CHIEF COMPLAINT
BRAIN TUMOR

CHIEF COMPLAINT
BRAIN TUMOR

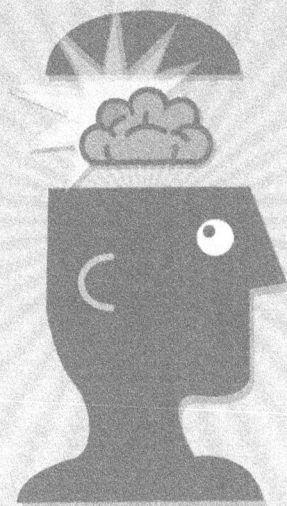

JOHN KERASTAS

SUNSTONE
PRESS

SANTA FE

Sunstone books may be purchased for educational, business, or sales promotional use.
For information please write: Special Markets Department, Sunstone Press,
P.O. Box 2321, Santa Fe, New Mexico 87504-2321.

Book design › Vicki Ahl
Cover design › Gerard Design
Body typeface › Palatino Linotype
Printed on acid-free paper
∞

———

Library of Congress Cataloging-in-Publication Data

Kerastas, John, 1953-
  Chief complaint : brain tumor / by John Kerastas.
    pages cm
  Includes bibliographical references.
  ISBN 978-0-86534-908-7 (softcover : alk. paper)
  1. Brain--Cancer--Popular works. I. Title.
  RC280.B7K386 2012
  616.99481--dc23

                        2012033257

———

WWW.SUNSTONEPRESS.COM
SUNSTONE PRESS / POST OFFICE BOX 2321 / SANTA FE, NM 87504-2321 /USA
(505) 988-4418 / ORDERS ONLY (800) 243-5644 / FAX (505) 988-1025

Dedication

TO MY FAMILY,
who have stood right beside me through my darkest days.

Contents

Acknowledgements

I HAVE MANY PEOPLE TO THANK for aiding me in my journey, my recovery and my recuperation. For starters, I need to thank my loving family including my wife, Barbara, son David, daughters Sara and Jennifer, brother Eric, sister Nancy and Mom and Dad.

My old college roommates (Jim Deline, Dick Lukey and Kurt Sands) reached out to me and gave me several well needed chuckles as well as encouragement.

I was very lucky to be ministered by Dr. Gail Rosseau, her extremely competent assistant Adrianna Valtierra, RN, and all the wonderful medical personnel and staff I encountered at the Evanston NorthShore Hospital.

In addition, there are numerous kind-hearted and patient folks who gave me hope and endured my antics during rehab especially Beth Sullivan and Violet Potocki, both first-rate rehab therapists.

I probably wouldn't have written this without the encouragement of Kathy Laya who gave me a terrific head start and numerous helpful tips.

I also received substantial encouragement from Greg Bliss, Alan Boyer, Rob Jackson, Lisa Machtemes, and Gary Poole.

The good folks from the First United Methodist Church of Evanston were outstanding in their support including Pastor Dean Francis, Deacon Jane Cheema, Pastor of Pastoral Care Bob Keller, Patricia Haughney, Mary Rawlinson and all my other Appalachia Service Project buddies.

Also, key to writing this tome was the pitchers of coffee I had with my buddies at Mrs. Dee's restaurant, i.e. Tom Gillespie, Dave Johnson and Marty Kohr, and probably a bunch of people I've forgotten.

My taste buds want to especially thank Phil Krone who cooked his absolutely delicious four leg, three bean chili for us (or was it four bean, three leg chili?) which seemed like manna from heaven.

Numerous work friends provided substantial motivational support including David Brochu, Tim Holtan, Bob Leah, Duane Martin, Bill Nieman and Steve Tonissen, among others.

I've gotten tremendous inspiration from the brain tumor community especially from bloggers and authors like Liz Holzemer, Samantha Kittle, Amy Marash, Kaylin Marie, and Beth Rosenthal.

I also am especially appreciative of James Clois Smith Jr., President of Sunstone Press for taking a chance on a previously unknown and unpublished author.

Lastly, I need to thank my old Burnett boss and mentor, Cynthia Stone, for her steadfast support and friendship through the years.

Preface

"Laughter is the best medicine"
—Unknown

The official *United Methodist Committee on Relief* presentation for training *Early Response Teams*[1] states that, "there are four emotional tasks for survivors in recovering from a disaster":

1. Accept the reality of the situation (I can't believe it happened).

2. Experience the pain (it's okay to hurt).

3. Accept that a new situation is required.

4. Withdrawing the emotional investment in the past and transferring it to the new.

1

"Chief Complaint: Brain Tumor"

"CHIEF COMPLAINT: BRAIN TUMOR," that was the subject line in the memo from my neurosurgeon to my general practitioner.

I did have a brain tumor. But the memo makes it sound like I knew I had a brain tumor and that it was just one of several complaints, "I have a sprained ankle, a sore back and can you do something about this brain tumor?" I want the record to show that I didn't even *know* that I had a brain tumor.

So, how do you know if you have a brain tumor? The clues aren't always obvious. According to the American Brain Tumor Association's (ABTA's) excellent website,[1] headaches are a common "initial symptom" for my type of brain tumor (meningioma). Headaches are also, well, common, and don't usually mean that you have a brain tumor.

Seizures are another indicator. If you have a seizure, it's pretty obvious that you need to go see a doctor.

But what if you don't have a headache or a seizure? I didn't.

Mental and personality changes are also a warning. While "mental changes" sounds ominous, they could be as innocuous as short-term memory problems, speech glitches or concentration lapses.

And while I had my share of "senior moments," none of them seemed any worse than the senior moments of my friends.

In the beginning, my chief complaint was that my eyesight was becoming wonky.

What do I mean? Well, in the summer of 2010, I began to recognize that something was wrong with my vision. On an erratic basis, in the right vertical third of my right eye, I would see a cascading series of irregular, amoeba-like images that looked like they were straight out of a petri dish. The rest of my right eye and my entire left eye saw what everybody else saw.

At first, I tried to ignore it. I told myself that it was a floater. It did, when it occurred, interrupt my train of thought but, as my friends and family will tell you, that isn't a particularly well-connected railroad in the first place.

Why didn't I run to the doctor when I first started seeing these wild images? Well, I have a tendency, and I suspect other folks do too, to put off learning about bad news, especially regarding health issues. This is, of course, irrational behavior. In almost every case, the earlier you know about a health problem the easier it is to fix.

So why pretend you don't have a health problem? It wasn't that I couldn't handle the truth; it was more like I didn't want to handle the truth right then. But even though I was in full denial, I knew I had to "pop the pimple" sooner than later.

I know people who, even when they know they have a serious health issue, avoid going to the doctor. My grandmother's sister refused to go to the doctor even though she was going blind. Guess what? She went blind.

I'm not sure, but I think we do this because we believe that if we can just hide from the bad news for a few more days (or weeks or months), it will buy us time. It will buy peace. It will buy calm before the impending storm. And maybe, just maybe, this aching back or sore throat or strange eye problem will fix itself.

Facing bad news head on takes some courage.

I knew a lady who summarized this saying, "You have to run to the fire." While she used it in a business context, it applies here as well. A burning problem won't go away on its own. It might not go away with the help of the best hospital or medical team in the world, but it can also turn into a forest fire if you don't ask the question, "What's wrong with me?"

I needed to ask that question.

But at the time I felt pretty healthy, and the thought of being seriously sick or ill just didn't make sense to me. I was training for the North Shore Century, a 100-mile bike ride, and a summer of training had made me feel pretty fit. On top of that, the year before I had run the Chicago "Rock 'n Roll" half-marathon with my youngest daughter, and later that year I finished in the top third of my age group in the Chicago Triathlon. I ate reasonably, wasn't overweight, and my cholesterol and other health indicators were on target. How could I, of all people, be sick? My hubris was about to be punctured and deflated like a bike tire running over a rusty nail: noisily, emphatically, and painfully.

I thought of my college roommate who had developed Stage II diabetes. Since my paternal grandfather had died from diabetes, I knew that this was serious stuff. The first time I saw my old roommate, after we had returned from a seven-year overseas assignment, I was shocked. In college he was, maybe, 215 lbs. or so. Since I'd last seen him, he had ballooned up to something north of 350 lbs. I couldn't figure out how this happened. In addition to putting on weight, he had lost all the feeling in his feet. He had broken a toe and hadn't noticed it until he looked down one day and said, "Gee, that toe isn't supposed to be at a right angle to my foot." (Actually, I'm pretty sure he didn't say "Gee.") And, here's the scary part: he's one of the smartest people I know… way smarter than I am.

I was determined and committed to being fit and staying healthy. So I ate "right," exercised and kept my weight close to my "race weight" (the weight I needed to be in order to meet my triathlon and biking goals).

How did I know that something was wrong, I mean really, disastrously wrong? Well, the strange visions I was experiencing, which I had initially ignored, were certainly a clue. It's the kind of clue that jumps up and down yelling, "Check me out, you dummy!"

But I was focused on my work. I continued to finish up a freelance marketing project and look for another consulting assignment. I yearned to be working at a start-up company with some spiffy new invention or intellectual property, or at some green technology company that was riding the wave of environmental investments. I couldn't wait to be flying around the country "with my hair on fire" visiting prospective clients, briefing analysts, and supporting sales cycles. Work was exciting, rejuvenating, and fulfilling.

Had I stopped and started a little self-examination, I might have pieced together some clues that, in hindsight, were pretty damn obvious. At the beginning of the year, for example, I started walking into a corner of our massive kitchen island with my right thigh—bam! It's a thick sheet of black granite with natural whorls and swirls that weighs a ton or two. So when you bang into it going full tilt towards the TV in the front room, it hurts. It's also hard to miss seeing—you could spread out a blanket and do a yoga lesson on the thing. I banged into it a number of times. So even though I never heard of anybody else just whacking the corner of their kitchen island with their hip on a fairly regular basis, I just passed it off as encroaching middle-aged feebleness.

More expensively, I started scraping the right side of my old ten-year-old black car against the inside of the white garage door. I quickly learned that the absolute minimum cost of fixing scrapes of that sort cost a grand, sometimes more. Since my car was black and the garage was white, the scrapes were pretty ugly and obnoxious. In addition to the money that was just plain wasted, I was disappointed in myself: how could I keep making the same mistake? I told myself that we had an old, tight garage door opening and that the ninety-degree turn from the alleyway took some mental acuity. Of course that didn't explain why, after years of pulling into the garage without a problem, all of a sudden I started scraping the car. It also didn't explain why my wife never scraped her car.

As the "man" of the family, I was the designated driver for almost every family excursion. Lately, however, I kept getting these little shrieks and tensed muscles from my wife when I drove. Geez, that was annoying. At the time, I had a good driver's record, no accidents for years. So, of course, I thought she was just getting older and more jittery—old age, you know? Looking back, I now realize that she probably had great reasons to close her eyes, wince and verbally jab me on my driving.

The thought that I just couldn't see well out of the lower right-hand corner of my eye was simply not something that ever occurred to me. Why? I don't know. The idea of going blind was just plain on the outside of the front door to my self-image, no matter how loudly my increasing blindness knocked, kicked and scraped to get in my consciousness.

In late August, though, I had one day where I saw these disconcerting and disconnected-from-reality amoebas five times. Even for me that seemed a bit excessive. So, of course, I waited until after the North Shore Century ride in early September to dial up my physician. My general practitioner did what any good GP does; he packed me off to an ophthalmologist.

So on Thursday, September 23, I went to see the ophthalmologist. My first impression of his office was that it looked like something straight out of a Swedish movie about unhappy people trapped in bland lives they didn't want to live. The waiting room added to that effect by displaying several abstract paintings in murky blues and purples that seemed to be drawn by patients with deep psychological issues.

I was nervous, so I thumped my fingers on the finely rendered Naugahyde chair until my name was called. I was shown into a room that looked like a set from the movie *The Silence of the Lambs*. It was outfitted with a machine that appeared to be designed for three-eyed aliens, and tools that looked like they belonged in a dentist's office. This, of course, did nothing to put me at ease.

The doctor looked very professional, complete with lab coat, country-club tie, and an expensive pen. He was indeterminately middle-aged, which is a good thing in doctors: too old and you worry that they've forgotten things; too young, and you worry that they haven't learned enough to forget.

I guess at this time I should confess that I am squeamish about my eyes. Watching my wife put in her contacts gives me the willies (the "willies" are a technical term for describing the feeling you get when your folks take you to a haunted house or scary roller-coaster ride about five years before you are emotionally ready to go). Her ability to touch her eyeball with her finger runs shivers up my spine. (I think she mostly does it to torment me.)

So I normally flunk the eye test where a technician touches your eye with a strange device that measures something important to keep you from developing some debilitating eye disease. Why do I flunk? Because I can't keep my eye open long enough for the doctor (or nurse or strong, hairy orderly) to get a measurement.

Ensconced in his clean, tidy, and vaguely sinister office, the doctor (I've repressed his name and most of the unsettling experience) told me that I needed to come back and see another doctor who specialized in a different but closely aligned field.

So the next week (in my mind there was no hurry), I visited this new doctor in the same somehow disquieting office. Here, a medical technician gave me a Visual Field test, essentially a fancy and, I suspect, expensive eye exam. In a Visual Field test, you look into a TV screen that makes you feel like you're viewing a bad, old-time sci-fi movie. Lights flash on and off in various areas, and you're supposed to click a button every time you see a light flash.

Apparently I flunked the test, or at least an important part of the test. How did I know? Because the doctor recommended that I have a magnetic resonance imaging ("MRI") test. For the uninitiated, MRI tests are normally scheduled for folks who have something lousy going on inside.

To take an MRI, you go to a lab hidden deep in some medical facility where they store the really high-powered medical equipment. Over in a corner you'll probably see a lab technician peering at a backlit green screen that reminds you of the sonar technology they must use on a nuclear submarine.

You are instructed to take off all your jewelry (this took about a nano-second) as the technician asks you questions like, "Do you have any metal in your body?" "Have you ever had a joint replacement using metal?" "Does being enclosed in very small space and having abnormally loud sounds clang and bang around your head drive you berserk?"

While I may be wrong, I think that no matter what your answer is, you are then told to lie down on a cloth-covered surfboard at a perpendicular angle to the MRI. It's so the technicians can easily slide you into the machine and bombard you with x-rays. I'm just guessing on the kind of rays, they could be beta rays for all I know. (Actually, I was hoping that they weren't beta rays because, as everybody who's ever worked in software knows, the "beta" version is pretty iffy stuff.) After you lie down, the technicians strap you down and quickly run out of the room. No, it isn't reassuring.

The machine started and the vibrations reminded me of some large ship leaving port. It began as a low hum that pulsed and shook. Abruptly, the promised clanging and banging commenced at erratic and irregular intervals. It felt as if something was really wrong with the machine, like maybe they forgot to add oil during the last seventy-five-thousand-mile overhaul or the thing needed new brake pads.

While I half-expected the MRI to explode or shoot me out the front like a torpedo, it didn't. And I walked away thinking, "Boy, I'll bet I won't have to do that again." Little did I know that I should've quickly joined the MRI frequent scanner club for the "points."

The MRI test was a bit unnerving. It was the first time I starting believing that maybe something was really wrong. When I got home, I took Louis for a walk. Louis was our half German shepherd, half Labrador, all lovable dog. We went for a walk almost every day I was in town. When I was in training for my triathlons, he ran along. When Barbara and I went for a walk, he came along. When I needed to be alone with my thoughts, he came along. I was never alone when he was around.

He was also a hunter. Any critter that dared to land, run or skitter across our yard was fair game. He chased squirrels, rabbits, chipmunks and caught some of each. He also caught a raccoon in our backyard and fought him to a draw (after which I took him to an emergency animal hospital for various stitches and shots). He loved us and we loved him.

Shortly afterwards, my wife Barbara and I went to the ophthalmologist's office to see the results of the MRI.

Barbara is a very steady soul to have with you at times like these. While she will yell and scream and turn red when the Chicago Bears have a dumb turnover or stupid penalty, she is relatively unflappable when somebody had a serious health issue. Growing up in the Detroit area, she paid her own way through college by working two jobs in the summer and working part-time jobs during the school year. Unlike me, she looks about ten years younger than she really is. She's an attentive mother, loves Project Runway, and eats less than most birds. We'd been married over thirty years and neither of us had yet had a major health problem.

The ride through the tree-lined streets of Chicago's north shore suburbs to the ophthalmologist's office, though, seemed longer that the four or five miles than it was. My memory of that ride was that we talked about everything except the reason for the ride—the nice fall weather, possible movies we should go to, and maybe the piles of leaves in the gutters above the third-floor attic.

But I knew that, this time, something was wrong, something that wouldn't be easily fixed. My fear was that I had some horrible eye problem that would require surgery. My parents had both had cataract surgery and it sounded unnerving.

So I stewed on the idea of eye surgery (What else could it possibly be?) during the drive and, in the process, torqued my nerves so tight that I would've needed a socket wrench to loosen them.

We took an elevator up to the ophthalmologist's office and, unlike previous visits, we were quickly shown into an examination room.

Almost immediately, the doctor entered the room and shut the door. Then in a no-nonsense tone of voice he told us that I had a brain tumor and he could recommend a very good neurosurgeon.

My tongue tied itself up, then slightly loosened, and I sputtered out something like, "brain tumor?"

I was stunned. I was shocked. I wasn't even sure what a brain tumor *was* other than bad, very bad.

What do you say to somebody who's just told you that your life is going to change, for the worse? "Thanks for the really bad news?" "Please excuse me while I start to freak out?" "Where's the scotch? And not the Black Label, I want the really good Blue Label stuff!"

I have no real memory of what was said other than some comment about sending me to a neurosurgeon that specializes in brain tumors.

There was a painful discontinuity about hearing life-changing news on an absolutely beautiful autumn day. The warm fall weather hadn't changed. The streets were teeming with students who just escaped from grade school. But I had just heard the worst news I could ever remember hearing. And the only people who knew it were me, my wife, and the ophthalmologist's medical team.

We had been referred to Dr. Gail Rosseau. Her online biography listed a stack of degrees, associations, and awards. According to a *Chicago Tribune* article, she had been on the President's short list for Surgeon General. Even without knowing that, her bio told us that she was what we needed. We scheduled an appointment for her earliest availability.

Dr. Rosseau's office was maybe ten to fifteen minutes away from our house. While it had the same vanilla furniture that the ophthalmologist's office had, the place bustled. Patients were zipping in and out. Nurses walked purposefully. The receptionist was awake and pleasant. These weren't characters out of an unhappy Swedish movie. These were medical practitioners with important work to be done. I felt reassured.

How does one describe Dr. Rosseau? I think the answer is with lots of adjectives and exclamation points. While physically, she's a short blond woman with impeccable taste, her presence is nearly overwhelming. She strides into the room, grabs your hand, and introduces herself with a strong, hardy voice: "I'm Gail Rosseau and we're going to take good care of you!" And if she didn't literally say that, I felt as though she had. She was strong. She was confident. She was everything you would ever want in somebody who would be cutting open your skull and scooping out a brain tumor. From that moment on, my wife and I have referred to her as "The Good Doctor."

She whisked us into a viewing room that had an entire wall which was backlit by some special medical lights. She set a large piece of sturdy medical film on an imitation wood railing. The film looked like an X-ray of a skull. In fact, it was my skull. Dr. Rosseau then said something like "See this big black area here, this is a brain tumor."

The black area looked like the biggest thing inside my head. This is commonly referred to as the "Oh, Shit" moment. You can't run away from it. You can't hide from it. It's there inside your head no matter where you go.

I mean, we all know on an intellectual level that we are mortal, but being shown that picture of a dark mass crushing the rest of my brain...well, it had the emotional impact of being hit with a sledgehammer. It hurt.

I don't remember much else about the meeting. She had a very competent assistant. They gave us some guidelines for the next few weeks prior to surgery. The bigger immediate issue, of course, was that now we had to tell everybody.

Brain tumors, in general, are not that common. According to the ABTA, "for every 100,000 people in the United states, approximately 209 are living following the diagnosis of a brain tumor." It's like the odds of winning a lottery scratch card, only this is a lottery you don't want to win. *The Good Doctor* believed that my tumor was a meningioma, which is pretty common in the world of brain tumors. Roughly 32% of all brain tumors are a meningioma. If you have to have a brain tumor, this is the one to have: it's slow-growing, benign (i.e., not cancerous), and rarely spreads to other parts of the body. Said differently, brain cancers are really, really, really bad. My meningioma tumor was merely bad.

The phrase "brain tumor" is scary and difficult to slide into any casual, over-the-fence-with-the-neighbor conversation. I imagined the following conversation when running into a friend at Starbuck's:

"Hey Fred, how's it going?"

"Great! Our daughter Mary just made the high school jazz band as the bass player, the only student to ever be picked as a sophomore."

"Congratulations!"

"And you, how's it going?"

"Well, I've just been diagnosed with a brain tumor—the tumor's as big as your wife's fist."

"No shit. Well...how about them Bears?"

And with your more competitive acquaintances, I could imagine the following conversation with Ashton:

"John, how are you? It's good to see you."

"I've just been diagnosed as having a brain tumor."

"Really, what kind?"

"It's a Grade I meningioma. It's about as big as your fist."

"Well, my brother Dave has a Grade III metastatic brain tumor. It's a Gliomas type of brain tumor. We're very worried about it infiltrating adjacent brain tissue. You should be grateful that you only have a Grade I meningioma!"

Aside from telling close family members personally, there are a whole slew of people who would want to know: business associates, close friends, and relatives. With that in mind, my socially perceptive wife suggested that we inform many of these people via email. Why? The deep-felt emotions that got conjured up every time we told somebody became onerous. Every conversation reminded us of how horrible the outcome could be.

With that in mind, my wife crafted an informative yet calming email about my condition. This is what it said:

Dear Friends,

I wanted to send you a quick note today to let you know of some surgery that John will be having this week. John had been experiencing some odd, random vision problems over the last couple of months, and finally went to have it checked out. An MRI finally revealed that his symptoms are the result of a slow growing brain tumor.

Now before you freak out...

The early diagnosis is good. The surgeon believes it is benign and has probably been there for some time, and is optimistic for a successful surgery and full recovery. John is in good shape and has not experienced any other symptoms, which also bodes well. But obviously, it is major surgery and John's recovery will probably take a few weeks.

Please forgive the email. We've both been finding it hard to tell people about this over the phone. But we wanted to let you know what was going on, and to ask that you keep John in your thoughts and prayers this week. Surgery is scheduled for Thursday, and I'll be sure to keep you posted.

We'll sure appreciate your positive thoughts this week—thanks.
Barb and John

As you can imagine, the responses to her email were thoughtful and considerate. For example:

Barb and John,
Thanks so much for letting us know. For certain, our thoughts will be with you this week and in the coming weeks.
We are so sorry to hear of this hurdle in your life, John, but relieved to hear that the prognosis is so positive. And as anyone can attest, you are a strong dude on several levels, so that will surely be a plus.
We'll be thinking of you and please keep us in the loop. And if there is anything we can do, please don't hesitate to let us know.
All the best, fondly,

And the following:

Hi Barb and John:
____ forwarded this email to me; I am sending prayers and positive thoughts to you. Please add my email to your list; I would love to know how you all are doing.
Much love and prayers.

And even this one from one of my old college roommates:

Hmmmm. 'Been there for some time' you say. Like back to the seventies on Lake Lansing Road [where our rental house was located]? I wondered what was going on in that brain sometimes.

I am, not to put too fine a point on it, a bit blunter. So I decided to send out a few emails of my own, like this one:

From: John Kerastas
Sent: Tuesday, October 26, 2010 2:30 PM
To: ____

Subject: For Your Eyes Only

I wanted to send you a short note telling you that I have a brain tumor and will be undergoing surgery on Thursday. More importantly, I want to thank you for all your support, direction and guidance over the years. You are a very special person and I wish you nothing but the best. John

Well, guess what kind of a reaction that got?

From: ____
To: John Kerastas
Sent: Oct 26, 2010 2:35 PM
Subject: RE: For Your Eyes Only
Oh, my God, John. What can I do to help? Please let me know…and tell your wife to keep me informed of your condition. I am here to help her and you. Please call on me. You are in my prayers. You helped me when I really, really needed it, and now I need to return the favor as well as I can. You are a strong and healthy character, John, so keep the faith.

I remember feeling really good about her reaction. She cared. My wife, though, made it clear in one of those non-verbal, part telepathic, feminine reactions that perhaps she should be the family spokesperson on my diagnosis and status moving forward.

The weekend before the surgery was beautiful. The autumn colors were in full bloom with vivid reds, oranges, and yellows decorating the northern suburbs of Chicago. The days were warm, the evenings cool and the air crisp. As luck would have it, we had tickets for the Michigan State versus Northwestern football game that Saturday, and one of my old college roommates, Kurt, came into town for the game.

Kurt, like me, is a big Michigan State fan. We had lived through the very lean (i.e. "losing") years while attending MSU, and were relishing the strong team they currently had. For Kurt to see a live game, however, was a bit unusual, but not for the reasons that you might normally think. Kurt was such a fan that he just couldn't bear to watch the Spartans lose. His solution? He taped every game and asked his wife to check the score and tell him whether he should watch the game or not. And, yes, he only watched games that MSU won. As a result, he hadn't watched anything but a taped game in years. The thought of watching a game in which they might lose, in addition to a troubling family issue of his own, added to his pre-game tension.

The night before the game, all three of us—Barbara, Kurt, and I—went to Bluestone, a local restaurant, for dinner. Bluestone is one of those great neighborhood restaurants. The meals are a congenial mixture of comfort food, kid food, and seafood. You can get a nice craft beer as well as a man-sized glass of red wine. The place was normally noisy and crowded on a Friday night, and the football crowd that night had just dialed all that up a notch or three.

Over refreshments, Barbara and I relayed our email stories to him. Barbara told him how she thought long and hard about how to tell everybody about my tumor without being alarming.

She paraphrased her note with characteristic clarity. She then mentioned a bit about my somewhat funereal email to my old boss.

Kurt's first words were something like: "You *didn't*, did you?"

"Yes, I did," I answered truthfully. "I sent her an email that thanked her for all her guidance and nurturing over the years, and implied that I expected to die from a brain tumor."

At first, he seemed a bit shocked. And then, I seem to remember him just putting his head between his two hands, looking down at the table, and laughing-for-crying as he shook his head while saying something like, "No, you didn't really do that...did you?"

And while Kurt had his family issue, and I had my tumor, the ice was broken. We imbibed. We laughed. We relaxed. We were now free to respond to the craziness of the situation and non-verbally say to ourselves, "Tonight we drink, for tomorrow we ride!" (This line is best said in a bad, old-western-film accent.)

And we did.

After the football game, we decided to grab a burger and a beer at a local restaurant. (MSU did win, but was down by a lot at the half, so a few refreshments were in order.) My son, David, and Kurt sat across from Barbara and me. After a glass of water (I was parched after all that yelling at the game), I excused myself for a trip to the restroom. Upon returning, I walked up to our booth and, looking at Kurt and David, said, "Where's Barbara?"

I remember hearing Barb's sweet voice say, "I'm right here." She laughed, thinking I was trying to make some sort of stupid joke. But the joke was on me. I couldn't see her, and she was only three feet from me sitting down at the table. It was then that I realized that I was partially blind. The tumor seemed to have knocked out the peripheral vision of my right eye.

Damn.

I sidled into my seat and tried to make some lame joke. I got the sense that this was a serious turn in the road that I ought to pay attention to, but I didn't really know how to react to it, what to do or when to do it.

The phrase "brain tumor" is big and scary to most everybody. There are good reasons for this, there's nothing about the words "brain tumor" that imply "good health" or "long life."

In addition, in case you repressed the heart-to-heart post-MRI discussion with your surgeon, the pre-surgery papers you sign make it absolutely clear that all bets are off. The surgeons will do their best, but there are lots of reasons, beyond their control, that really bad things can happen once they cut open your skull.

From what I can tell, most folks react in one of three ways:

Obsessing about it
Pretending it isn't happening
Becoming an amateur expert on brain tumors

Let's take a quick look at these obvious but, in my opinion, flawed emotional responses.

Obsessing about it

This is the most natural and immediate response. "Ohmigod, I have this thing growing inside my head and it's going to kill me!" While this may be true, it doesn't seem to help anything. You may find some sort of temporary tension release by making everybody around you crazy, but they may just strangle you before the operation.

In that vein, I imagined this conversation with my deceased, no-nonsense aunt.

"Aunt Ann, I have this big, scary tumor and I could die."

"Well dear, it's time to take this like a big boy. After all, you are 57 years old."

"But, Aunt Ann, the idea of a big tumor in my brain gives me the willies!"

"Now John, while we're all sorry about this, you are becoming rather tiresome."

"But I could die."

"Well, if that shuts you up, then please hurry up about it."

Pretending it isn't happening

When I was in high school and had what I was sure was terminal acne, pretending that I didn't have acne just didn't work. For example, I'd walk up to some girl in the hallway and say: "Linda, isn't trigonometry tough enough without Mrs. Butler giving us five pages of problems every night?"

Her reply: "John, your zits are disgusting."

Now, the analogy doesn't quite work when you have a brain tumor because, unless she's Supergirl and has X-ray vision, she won't know that you have a brain tumor. (Actually, she might need MRI-vision to really appreciate the tumor.)

Whether you acknowledge your problem or not, I don't know of any serious issue that gets "better" if you ignore it.

President Kennedy: "Robert, if we ignore the Russian missiles in Cuba, will this whole thing just blow over?"

Robert Kennedy: "John, 'blow over' could turn into 'blow up' if we don't do something."

Here are some other problems that have gone to hell in a hand basket while I pretended things weren't that bad:

My 401k certainly didn't fix itself while the economy decided to dive into the nearest mineshaft.

Ignoring my inability to hit a jump shot didn't help me make the junior high basketball team (by the time I hit senior high school, I knew better than to try out).

Sitting on the sidelines while I watched interest rates collapse didn't make my mortgage payments go down.

As best I can tell, problems only get worse, not better, the longer you ignore them.

Becoming the leading amateur expert on brain tumors

Soon after discovering that I had a brain tumor (about a minute after I got home), I logged onto the excellent ABTA website to better understand what a brain tumor was, and what my chances of surviving might be.

And while all signs pointed to me having a Grade I meningioma tumor, nobody really knew for sure what I had until they took a saber saw to my skull and peered inside. Okay, it wasn't a saber saw; in good hospitals most operations are done with radial arm saws. (Personally, I recommend the 10" Sears Craftsman, 3-horsepower radial arm saw with LaserTrac.)

In any case, my research revealed that I could possibly have another type of tumor, many of which can start to infiltrate surrounding tissue. On top of that, the experts consistently warn patients that "your tumor is unique and might not conform to the 'average' characteristics described."

Well, that sounded ominous. Does that mean my meningioma might decide one day to start infiltrating my brain instead of just having a lovely time tap dancing in the tissue between my brain and my skull?

The more I learned, the more nervous and upset I got. So I just stopped reading.

Now, this won't work for everybody. My son and sister became resident experts on the potential types of tumors, treatments, and worst-possible-case scenarios. They are also smarter than I am, have lots of degrees, and don't mind reading sixteen-letter words like Oglioastrocytoma (this is a particularly nasty tumor—see the ABTA website for details).

So how did I becalm the nasty thoughts emanating from the reality of a brain tumor?

Humor. Black Humor. Sophomoric Humor. Sophomorically Black Humor.

Said differently, if I didn't have Black Humor, I wouldn't have any humor at all. Actually, Ray Charles said it better in his song titled, *If it Wasn't for Bad Luck*. Maybe a better analogy is *Life is Beautiful* by Roberto Benigni, because for me the only way for me to cope with this depressing situation was to find the humor in having a tumor.

So, much to the chagrin of my doctors, nurses, orderlies, and, yes, often my wife, I used gallows humor to mask my uneasiness, my concerns, and my nerves.

Now, for starters, medical professionals of all shapes and sizes often mention that some patients like to name their tumors. Somehow, I couldn't wrap my mind (so to speak) around the idea. While I can rationally understand that putting a name to some unknown and dangerous opponent both demystifies and dulls it, I had trouble finding the right name.

Here's what I considered:

Darth Vader—too cartoonish, plus you always knew he would lose in the end... and the end was still TBD for me.

Dr. H.H. Holmes? He is the villain in Erik Larson's book, *The Devil and the White City*, and way too scary. I think he still scares the author.

Perry the Parasite—a bit childish, but this came closer to how I felt about my tumor. It was feeding off my blood in order to grow. Which, of course, led to—The Vampire Tumor—this gave me visions of Bela Lugosi, who scared the snot out of me as a child. And, I'm too old to get into *The Twilight Saga*. Besides, I hear that they turn away anybody who's over 30 at the movie theater.

The Blob! For those of you too young to remember, *The Blob* is a horror/science fiction film from the 1950s that depicts a giant amoeba-like alien that lives by consuming (absorbing?) humans and growing ever larger. While I've never formally named my tumor, the name *The Blob* best captured the emotional landscape of my feelings about my tumor.

So I gave up on coming up with a name for my tumor. I decided instead to turn to—yes, you probably guessed it—American musical theater to demystify and express my inner feelings about *The Blob* in my brain. So here it is (sung to the tune of "Oklahoma," with apologies to Rodgers and Hammerstein):

Meningioma
Where a tumor grows rampant in my brain
Where my suffering head
Fights slow growing cells
In my precious arachnoid mater.

Meningioma
Where my tumor's really quite large
While benign and slow
Has continuous growth
And those vicious cells squash my brain.

We snip it and throw it in the trash
And my brain is alone AT LAST.

And when I say hey! A yippy-i-o-ey
I'm only saying you're a pain Meningioma
Meningioma M-E-N-I-N-G-I-O-M-A
Meningioma, Not Okay!

I sent the lyrics to my family for review. The kinder-hearted ones made gentle "how interesting" noises. But I'm sure they started to ask themselves, "How deep has this thing penetrated?"

Since I was mentally preparing myself for the worst-case scenario (i.e. dying), I decided to be a man about it, and put my affairs in order. Affairs? What affairs? For the record, I want to state that I have never had an affair, have never tried to have an affair, and, can't imagine anybody wanting to have an affair with me. To this day, I'm shocked that my wife said "yes" when I asked her to marry me. And yes, I am happy to admit that *I Married Up* (cue the Antsy McClain song, and if you don't have it you can easily find it on YouTube).

As with most everything in life, I started the project by doing a little internet research and found out that I needed to: a) have a will, b) have a living will (which, strangely, is different), and c) tell my wife where our savings are stashed (including the silver dollars I keep in a coffee can by the workbench).

If I learned one thing in the process of writing a will: "Will" is easy to spell, but not so easy to write.

First you have to decide who gets what. You might decide that "if I'm dead, what do I care?" But if you do care about those you'll leave behind, you need one. Why? A will gives everybody somebody to blame when you're gone.

Well, that's easy, I thought. I'll just leave everything to my wife. Then I thought about my brother and my sister.

My brother, Eric, makes Jack Black look like an introvert. He's shorter than me, tons stronger, and an irrepressible optimist. While I have a classic Croatian build (tallish, thin), my brother could credibly do ads for the Ireland or Scotland tourist bureaus. No matter the time of year in Michigan, he's the guy wearing a Hawaiian shirt. More importantly, he's the rare single father of three overly active children and always seems to be in constant motion.

Given all that, his job is a huge stress-factor, and he has to think twice about every dollar he spends. And he appears to be relying on his company pension plan for his retirement. Okay, yes, I know. Have your laugh, take a deep breath and put your glasses back on.

He could certainly use a few extra pesos to pay the heating bills in the frigid Detroit area; shouldn't I give him a small slice of the Kerastas pie?

But if I leave $$$ for him (or even $), I'd have to include my sister, Nancy. She has even less savings than he does, and only a small pension from the State of Tennessee. Why? Well for starters, she has a Bachelor's Degree, a law degree, and a Doctor of Oriental Medicine degree. All those dang degrees all cost mucho buckaroos. On top of that, while her current position sounds exotic (she's an acupuncturist on a cruise ship traveling to exotic locations all over the world), she doesn't get paid much. And if that wasn't enough, she's the moral compass of the family. She has an unerring sense of right and will not tolerate wrong (e.g., she reports all her tips on her tax return). Now normally, that would make somebody absolutely intolerable. You'd smirk, chortle, and roll your eyes at everything that person does.

But she softens all that with one of the world's great giggles, an impish smile, and an infectiously caring interest in everybody else. So don't I need to leave her something, too?

Wait a minute, all my kids are living and my folks also are squeaking by on my Dad's pension.

This is just too complicated, so I left it all to Barbara. She will know what to do. And if all else fails, I figure she can take our hard-earned savings, find herself a good-looking gigolo, and enjoy herself.

There's also this little issue in the will about where you want to be buried. It seems like whenever we go visit my wife's relatives in Pennsylvania, a trip to the cemetery seems like a mandatory part of the itinerary. My wife's cousin takes us to the Catholic cemetery where all the PA relatives are buried. It's a nice cemetery just outside the small town of Derry. The grounds are a plushy green with a good view of the local valley.

The family plots are close enough to each other so that you can visit a bunch of graves in a short walk. The last time we went was really quite pleasant. So the idea of having one's remains close to the ones you love has a certain appeal.

But I had no idea if my family had a family plot, and where it is...or if Barb's family had a family plot. The questions started to mount.

On top of that, my wife is Catholic and I'm Methodist. Would her family's cemetery let me in? On the other hand, I'm pretty sure that Pastor Dean² wouldn't give a rat's ass if Barbara was buried next to me in a Methodist cemetery. Methodists are losing so many followers that you can probably join us even if you're deceased (I am also unconvinced that Methodists have the funds to have their own cemetery, at least those of us living above the Mason-Dixon Line).

I asked my Dad about a possible family plot or cemetery. Since he's the family historian, I thought he'd know. He did some digging and discovered that his mother and father are buried in the Detroit area. Their plot used to be in the middle of a calm and charming cemetery. Since being buried, however, the local cemetery sold an unused section of land to the local municipality to build a road. So, my grandparents' plots are on the edge of a rather busy road that has clouds of car exhaust wafting over it. It just doesn't sound like the place I want to be planted for eternity.

Now having a gravestone can be cool. I remember visiting Jim Morrison's grave in Paris and it seemed like every third visitor to the cemetery was humming a Doors tune.

But the greenie in me wonders about taking all that space for, essentially, memories. So I decided to sign up to be cremated. My will asks my survivors to spread half of my ashes on the MSU Marching Band practice field; and the other half on Mount Fuji. Since my college days and overseas business assignment in Japan are two of the favorite times in my life, this will give my family an excuse to see a football game and drink some really good sake. (Personally, I believe that sake is best enjoyed "hot" in an artfully crafted dish after a brisk walk in cold weather through a Japanese garden.)

The living will is designed to have you give direction to your family if, for reasons you don't really want to contemplate, you become incapable of giving it yourself.

And while I'd like to grow old, I don't want to lie in a bed with a beating heart but no light on in the attic. So I've asked my family to pull the plug when the downhill side has slid beyond the time when I'm recognizably "me."

How do you know when that's happened? Beats me! I still get teary over putting our cat down.

There's a scene in the movie *Ghost* where a couple wants Oda Mae Brown (Whoopi Goldberg) to talk to a deceased relative about an insurance policy that's missing. After I'm dead and gone, I don't want some gypsy woman in heavy make-up with an eastern European accent waking me up and asking me, "Where's the insurance policy?"

So I did two things. First, I organized all our investment records into an easy-to-read binder so that Barbara could figure out how to pay the bills should something bad happen. Given my bookkeeping, this was long overdue and harder than it should have been. I also showed Barbara where it all was so she didn't have to hire a detective.

I then organized a brief meeting with our financial advisor. I explained my situation to him and, not surprisingly, he was both sensitive and professional in reviewing where we stood. I tried to paint a "post-John" financial planning picture that would exclude gold mines in Bolivia and provide Barbara a picture of what funds she has available to her when she decides to retire.

I then felt that I could go into the operation with a clear conscience, if not a clear mind (I thought I'd say that before you did).

2

Welcome to the Hospital (the First Time)

THE DAY BEFORE MY OPERATION WAS GORGEOUS: sunny and Indian Summer warm. It evoked memories of Halloween, fresh-baked pies and football games. On the North Shore where we live, almost every street is lined with old trees, and our neighborhood is flooded with towering oak, maple, and black walnut trees. As this was late October, many of the leaves had fallen, creating a nicely messy mix of colored leaves on lawns, sidewalks and streets.

My son, David, decided to keep me company that day. Physically, David looks like the middle-distance runner he was in high school, a "tall drink of water." Personality-wise, he has all the attributes of a first-born male child: serious, task-oriented and independent. And, like me, food is never far from his thoughts.

After a morning's spin class at the gym, he offered to take me to what is reputed to be the best burger joint in the Chicago area, Kuma's Corner (to get a feel for the place, read the unapologetic home page of their website).

I can only describe the place as a head-bangers bar-cum-restaurant. It's the kind of place where sandwiches have names like "Black Sabbath," "Slayer," and "Iron Maiden." When I looked at the crowd, I got the feeling that the place had a three-tattoo minimum, so I was almost surprised when they let me in without a strange look or smirk.

The burgers were delicious. They were also large. When I say "large," I mean large for a steel worker, large for a professional football player, large for a Japanese family of four. I felt full after the first three bites. Not wanting to embarrass myself in front of my son, I kept at it. Bite by bite, I'd murmur things like "Mmmm good," "Don't want to rush this," and "Oh, momma."

We waddled out of the restaurant mid-afternoon and I was ready to go to sleep. It was the heaviest meal and the most meat that I could ever remember eating.

Little did I know that this burger would come back to haunt me.

Evanston NorthShore Hospital, where I was scheduled to have my surgery, is a first-class hospital just up the road from Northwestern University's lakeshore campus. Nestled into an area between a nicely kept up older neighborhood and a local par-three golf course, the hospital is surrounded by old big trees, dense bushes and green grass. The hospital building itself completed a major renovation not that long ago; and is clean, modern, and well kept. It's also busy. The lobby positively bustles with patients, families, doctors and technicians walking in and out and about.

It also seems right-sized. It's large enough to house a full range of doctors and experts without seeming to be as big and overwhelming as the Pentagon or the Merchandise Mart (a Chicago building that used to be the biggest building in the world). All in all, if you have to have surgery, it seems like a good place to be.

As best I can tell, the doctors at Evanston NorthShore hospital are not night owls. They like to have operations early in the morning. So my entourage (Barbara, son David, daughters Sara and Jenny) went with me to the hospital at the crack of dawn.

The day before the operation, I started to wonder about what to bring with me to the hospital. Oddly, the pre-operation briefing notes from the hospital warned you not to bring anything of value, which knocked out my iShuffle and laptop. It also made me vaguely uneasy. What kind of place is this that I have to be worried about thieves?

As an afterthought I threw in a book, *The Guernsey Literary and Potato Peel Pie Society,* which my wife recommended. I also grabbed some newspaper Sudoku puzzles with the vague thought that maybe I'd need to brush up on my mental fitness a bit after surgery.

My room, much to my relief, was private. I stowed my stuff in the closet. I walked around and noticed that if I stood up by the window I had a nice view of the Baha'i Temple (a strikingly beautiful building and local landmark). Then we started to wait.

I put on my flimsy robe. I fidgeted. We talked about the Spartans and their strong early start to the Big Ten football season. We made pithy remarks about the weather. David and I reviewed our Kuma burgers for the girls.

Much like the lead-up to my visit with the ophthalmologist, we talked about everything but the "elephant in the room": my brain tumor and my impending operation.

Finally, somebody came in to start up an IV. At one time, post-operation, I had three different IVs in me: one in the top of my right hand, one in the bottom of my right hand and one in my left hand. And while they may have looked icky, mine didn't really hurt.

In medical terms, I was going to have a craniotomy. A craniotomy is any bony opening that is cut into the skull. A section of the skull, called a bone flap, is removed to so that the surgeon can start working on the tumor underneath. Craniotomies come in all shapes and sizes: big ones, small ones and ones located all over the brain in inconvenient places or, as blogger Christie Clough Bishop puts it, "An Inconvenient Tumor...but aren't they all?"

The Blob, according to a memo from *The Good Doctor*, was located in "the superior sagittal sinus in the posterior parietal-Occipital region," which meant that the tumor was in the back of my skull towards the left-hand side. The plan, as I understood it, was to cut open my head, take out the tumor and glue the skull back, much like a jigsaw piece. As you can see, I had a rather simplistic understanding of what was about to happen.

I have bare shreds of memories of the operating room. The drugs kicked in quickly and quite effectively. I later learned that the drugs were so strong that I was put on a ventilator for the operation because I wouldn't have been able to breathe by myself. I'm glad I didn't know about that before the surgery.

I wasn't much help during the operation. I wasn't awake and being asked to move my arms or feet like some brain surgery patients. Suzy Becker in her book, *I Had Brain Surgery, What's Your Excuse?* talks eloquently about being awake during her brain operation and I shiver every time I think about it.

Speaking of not being much help, my sister told me a story about one of the top doctors of oriental medicine she's met. He apparently told a patient that the upcoming procedures were going to be very difficult. The patient choked out something like "Difficult? What do you mean?" The doctor answered, "Not for you, for me! You just lie there."

I laid on the operating table for six and a half hours. I'm not sure what the original estimate was for, but I think that was about twice as long as we thought it would be. Why that long? As *The Good Doctor* said afterwards, "I have plenty of respect for that tumor — it was a big, nasty one."

Hmmmm, that didn't sound so good.

I later learned that she decided not to cut out the entire tumor because she was afraid that if she cut through any more blood vessels, I would have had a stroke.

Hmmmm, that didn't sound so good, either.

She then told us that she took out about 70% of the tumor. What about the other 30%? In nearly the same breath, *The Good Doctor* mentioned that she'd get the rest of the tumor with radiation in three months or so.

Radiation? That sounded difficult, dangerous and a tad desperate. But, *The Good Doctor's* confident smile and disarming tone of voice put me at ease. She didn't seem alarmed. If she was fine, I guessed I would be fine.

I also learned that my tumor was, indeed, benign, and that I had two blood transfusions during the operation. I didn't tell my Dad because he's always worried that you might catch some horrible disease from a blood transfusion. I just kept wondering if that meant that I'd end up with thoughts from somebody else like they do in the CSI TV show (but it never happened).

I would later learn that a benign tumor doesn't mean "no problems." Meningioma can devastate lives in ways I never expected from a *benign* tumor. I learned all about this in great detail some days later when I later found and joined the terrific *It's Just Benign* website.

Soon after I awoke, my family swarmed into my room in the intensive care unit, congratulated me, and wished me all the best. I showed them my railroad tie-sized stitches, and they made appropriate "Ooooh-ing" noises. I think I got a tasty post-operation meal of Jello, beef broth and apple juice.

At the time, I felt pretty darn good. Little did I understand that I was so full of really powerful drugs that I wouldn't know if I were punched or stamped.

My family had a very different reaction to their first sight of me. My son told me that: "Physically, you looked like you'd been hit by a truck. You were extremely sluggish and weak, barely able to move, and I remember your voice being hoarse and low like you had a cold. Your sense of humor was like your normal sense of humor on steroids. You were cracking tons of jokes, but they were such extreme versions of your usual sarcasm that they sounded very strange to normal ears. At first it seemed like a new personality, but after talking with you for a while, we recognized you more. I imagine it's what you'd act like if you had ten beers in a sitting."

My youngest daughter was quite disturbed by it. She asked Barb, "Why is he acting like that?" And, of course, Barb reassured her, "He's full of drugs, honey."

After everybody left that evening, around 10 p.m. or so, I tried to get to sleep. For starters, the nurses had put some "calf-squeezers" (my words, not theirs) on my legs. These calf-squeezers would, now, take a wild guess, squeeze your calves every minute or so. I understand that this helps diminish problems with blood clots, which is a very good thing. At the same time, it's a strange and unusual sensation. Since nobody, not even Barbara, squeezes my calves through the night, it made sleep, well, challenging.

And, as I soon found out, patients in the Intensive Care Unit ("ICU") are not allowed to remove calf-squeezers by themselves.

Since I was on a drip IV to keep me well-hydrated, I felt a strong urge to go "#1" numerous times during the night. So the night nurse demonstrated how easy and convenient it was for me to use the little bedside bottle they provide for exactly that purpose. Apparently she thought that I needed the remedial instructions they provide to the particularly dull patients.

Now when it comes to peeing, I feel like I'm a baseball utility player in that I can contribute in lots of ways. I can pee in the woods, say on a camping trip. I can pee standing up. I can pee sitting down. I can even pee into a Japanese toilet (your aim has to be a bit better than usual).

But I can't pee in bed. I suspect it goes back to some severe training I received as a child.

I mentioned my disinterest in using the bottle to *Nurse Don't-Bother-Me* (I forgot her real name) and got a meaningful stare. Now, I'm not always accused of being the brightest bulb in the socket, and since I just had brain surgery, one might expect me to miss this message, but even I got it loud and clear: *Nurse Don't-Bother-Me* didn't want to be bothered, which is how I learned that ICU patients, especially those who just had brain surgery, are not allowed to go to the bathroom by themselves.

In my defense, I must say that I don't remember anybody telling me that I *couldn't* go to the bathroom by myself.

Now there are very, very good reasons why patients, especially those who have just had brain surgery, shouldn't get up and start walking around on their own. Those reasons mostly have to do with falling down and undoing all the surgery that patients, such as myself, just went through for six and a half hours earlier that day.

I, in my drug-addled state, thought, "I can walk to the bathroom by myself—it's only three, maybe four feet away."

So I ripped my legs out of the calf-squeezers (I soon came to think of them as shackles), swung my legs over to the side, repositioned my IV and started to get out of bed.

That's when all hell broke loose. Sirens went off. Lights Flashed. I heard the pounding of feet running (well, maybe a fast walk) coming towards my room. *Nurse Don't-Bother-Me* appeared. She explained that I was not allowed to get out of bed by myself and that I was a bad boy. This was delivered in a tone of voice reserved for dogs that had an accident on the living room floor.

Now's a pretty good time to fess up that one of my (many) faults is that I can get a bit sarcastic when somebody confronts me. My comments can range from sardonic to acerbic to caustic.

I find it truly amazing that I swallowed my instincts and said I'd follow this (new to me) rule moving forward. I still, however, needed to visit the necessary room.

Nurse Don't-Bother-Me wanted to watch to make sure I didn't fall down. I guess I'm stating the obvious when I say that, at least for a 57-year-old man, there is nothing about peeing that gets easier when you are tense and upset. And, for me, having a woman watch me pee is not relaxing. It felt like a dirty and unnecessary invasion of my privacy.

But here I was in this "Catch-22": I felt a strong urge to relieve my bladder, but couldn't due to being stressed out by the confrontation. Yet, I wasn't allowed to pee except *in Nurse Don't-Bother-Me's* presence. I'm sure she was wondering why I made such a fuss about getting up to pee, and then wasn't doing anything.

I explained that it was upsetting to have somebody watch me pee. A few seconds (minutes?) ticked by.

Nurse Don't-Bother-Me exclaimed that it was hospital policy to make sure us patients were safe. A few more seconds dragged by.

We then started a negotiation that was almost as tricky and laborious as the Paris Peace talks. Since I had to "go" I was at a significant disadvantage in the negotiations. Finally, we agreed that I was allowed to shut the door almost all the way, which did the trick and I went.

I'm sure she peeked.

At 2:30 a.m. or so, I was not a happy camper. I was upset that I couldn't go to the bathroom without somebody watching me. I wasn't happy that I still had more than a bit of Blob in me and the drugs made me feel like I'd just drunk five bottles of "5-Hour Energy." I was almost ready to ask for a seat belt, because I felt like I might just vibrate myself out of the bed and onto the floor.

Then I looked at the window. For some strange reason, the silhouette of the Baha'i Temple created a shadow that poured into my room. It seemed like there was something about the double-paned glass than enabled me to see it from my bed which, the more I thought about it, made no sense at all.

Since my room on the fifth floor was South and a little East of the Temple, I couldn't figure out how or why I would be able to see it. But there it was, larger than life, pouring into my room. And while it sounds silly and airy fairy, it was peaceful, it was calming, and it was holy. Here was tangible evidence that somebody (something?) was here with me in the dead of night.

As a lifetime Methodist, this is some confession and a somewhat disturbing one at that.

Since looking at the shadow of the Baha'i Temple calmed my nerves a bit, and I couldn't sleep, I turned on the light and decided that this was the perfect time for a little self-improvement. So I reached for the *Chicago Tribune* to tackle the day's Sudoku puzzle.

In hindsight, maybe this wasn't one of my better ideas, but at the time, I thought it'd give my brain something to focus on. I grabbed a pencil, found the puzzle and started in. After a few minutes to calibrate my thoughts, I thought I knew an answer to a square in the middle of the puzzle. I went to write a "2" in the middle-right box and my pencil landed in the box to the left of that.

That's funny. I tried it again, and again I missed the square entirely. Well now, this might be a bit tougher than I thought. I tried again. And this time I used by left had to guide my right hand into the correct square to write a "2." The "2" that I drew covered three, maybe four squares. Oops.

I tried to figure out the answer to another box. I studied the given numbers, extrapolated possible answers, and postulated possibilities. None of them made any sense. How could this be? I used to be able to do a level "3" Sudoku puzzle almost all the time. This was only a level "2," I should be able to breeze through this. I thought some more. I strategized. I figured. After a while, I figured out that I couldn't figure it out. Okay, maybe I can read.

So I picked up the book that my wife had recommended. I tried to read the first chapter and forgot which character was doing what to whom.

I reread the chapter, and moved onto the second, third and fourth chapters (maybe more). I got confused. Who was the heroine? What was the name of the farmer on the island? Why had the heroine started writing to this farmer? I started to keep notes on the plot; however, my handwriting was so bad that I couldn't read my own writing (I got a D-minus in handwriting in the third grade and, no, it hasn't affected me...much).

I have this vague memory of the story having an interesting romance, a strong, if flawed, hero, and an interesting setting.

I couldn't stomach any of that. I was in a dark, dark place, and anything that hinted of "sweetness" turned my stomach.

At about 3 a.m., I gave up and turned on the TV. This is when I became addicted to HGTV. I watched:

Design on a Dime
House Hunters
House Hunters International
American Pickers
Holmes on Homes
Color Splash
And anything else they showed.

I watched HGTV until the kitchen opened and I could order, whoopee, some more green Jello. I survived the first night.

That morning I had an idea on how to address my fears about being partially blind. The idea? To embrace a visual identity that would acknowledge my handicap while disarming it by making my blindness a badge of distinction.

I guess this is where I need to confess that, yes, I worked in advertising for twenty years. I'm not proud of it, but I can't deny it.

And, as it turns out, the most famous partially blind advertising guy was a well-dressed rogue in a Hathaway shirt ad. The ad features a man wearing a patch over one eye, standing up with a hand on one hip as he is being fitted for suit pants. The ad dramatically increased sales and made advertising history (search for "Hathaway Shirt ad" online and you'll find it). So I decided to make the one-eyed rogue my visual signature, my avatar if you will. To do so, though, I needed an accomplice, somebody who had access to a computer.

My nurse on the day shift was very nice, attentive without being overbearing. All she wanted to know was (1) if I was "comfortable," and (2) if I had gone "#2."

That dang Kuma burger hadn't yet shown up, and since I was really hoping to avoid an enema, I quickly changed the subject and asked her to help me with my Hathaway shirt campaign search. Since this request didn't seem within the normal bounds of the nurse-patient relationship, I felt that I needed to explain why finding and printing a picture of the infamous Hathaway shirt campaign[i] would help my recovery. So I started a conversation with my very nice nurse.

"I understand that patients with a positive attitude get healthier faster than those with negative attitudes."

"Yes, that's right."

"And you probably also heard that the tumor left me with a vision problem." (This was my play for sympathy.)

"Yessss?"

"I need your help in confronting this issue head-on."

"Okay, what do you want?"

Trying to sound as sincere as I could, I said "I want to confront my blindness by embracing it and even celebrating it a bit. I want to show the world, and myself, that I can cope with this little setback. How am I going to do that? This is where I need your help. I want to get a copy of the famous 'Man in the Hathaway Shirt' ad and tape it to the wall above my bed. That way everybody will understand my positive, if flippant, attitude about my blindness. It would mean a great, great deal to me. Will you help me?"

"John, your zits are disgusting."

"But will you help me?"

"Okayyyyy."

Being the understanding and compassionate nurse that she was, she went online and printed out a copy for me. Later that day, when my family and friends trooped into my room, I had the copy of the ad taped to the wall behind my bed. And, of course, only my wife (who was still in advertising) understood what that weird ad was about.

> To: Friends of all shapes and sizes
> Subject: Kerastas Update
> Date: Thu, 28 Oct 2010 20:13:10 -0500
>
> Hello all!
>   Wanted to send you a brief update on John's surgery today. It was long (6 1/2 hours!) but went well. He's resting in the ICU, wiggling fingers and toes, and talking—even cracking jokes and making sarcastic comments. He should be out of the ICU and in a regular room on Friday, providing everything continues to go well. Guessing he will be here recovering for a few days yet.
>   Wondering if I'm going to let him watch the Michigan State vs. Iowa football game on Saturday.
>   Thanks for all the thoughts, prayers and positive energy!
> Barb and John, David, Sara and Jenny"

In case you received this and were wondering, I didn't write this. The dead giveaway was that it was coherent and grammatically sound.

Strangely enough, a hospital is a hard place to get some rest, especially during the day. Why? Because everybody and I mean *everybody*, feels like they can walk into your room at any time.

"Sorry, Mr. Kerastas," without really meaning it, blurted the guy that came around every morning at 5 a.m just to peer in my eye and make sure I was alive.

"Time to change your IV." In bustles a nurse.

"Has your bed been made yet?" A nurse's assistant strolls in.

"Time for your vitals." Ditto.

"Has somebody checked your stitches?" In pops a resident.

"Have you ordered breakfast? Lunch? Dinner?" In comes the waitress (dressed in a spiffy tuxedo, I must add).

"How about your pills? Want some water?" (Now in my opinion, everybody has a unique skill that they are, or should be, proud of. Mine is being able to swallow pills *without* a glass of water—pretty impressive, huh?)

"Time for physical therapy."

"Time for occupational therapy."

"Can I clean your room?"

"Have you gone #2 yet? Want a stool softener?" I answered "no" and "yes."

"You have a visitor."

Now don't get me wrong, I needed and appreciated all this. It just made the days rather busy and somewhat noisy.

The hospital at night was totally different: quieter, darker, and more somber. And while nurses came waltzing into my room for vitals every other hour or so, that was about it. If you were an insomniac like me—hoping to go to sleep, wishing you could sleep, wondering why you couldn't sleep—the hospital at night was, well, a bit eerie.

My shackles still squeezed me. My Papa Bear-sized stitches were a bother. They made it hard to sleep on my back because they would jab into other parts of my head when I lay on my back. And the drugs seemed to course through my veins giving me a jolt every time some timed-release dosage kicked in. Around 2 a.m. or so, I started to hear the alarm notifying the staff of a patient out of bed without permission.

Wang. Wang. Wang.

The patient's voice was harsh and angry. "Why are you watching me go to the bathroom? I want some privacy!"

I remember the nurse (not Nurse Don't-Bother-Me) being quite calm, "You need to call us when you want to get up for your own safety."

This seemed to be happening right next door to me. I don't remember his retorts exactly, but he was angry, and getting angrier. "Leave me alone! And don't watch me going to the bathroom!"

I wish I could remember her exact words, but she simply said something like, "You need to get back into bed; you've just had a major operation."

He turned on her in a loud, ugly, strident tone of voice. "Go away, I don't want your help, leave me alone!"

The whole floor could hear the argument and the combative tone. I could hear footsteps racing down the hallway.

He then got even madder, yelled something like, "You fuckin' bitch! Who is in charge of this place? I've never been treated so badly in my entire life."

She was unbelievably restrained. "Now you need to get back into your room and get in bed, you can hurt yourself."

I could hear a little crowd surrounding him outside my door, blocking off his getaway lanes.

Then he screamed. It was a primeval scream of frustration and rage. It was the kind of scream that strained every vocal cord he had. It was the kind of scream that guys make just before they throw that first punch, "I've just had brain surgery and I CAN"T SLEEP."

Now this made no sense to me. He's just had brain surgery and the big reason he's upset is that he can't get to sleep? All he had to do is ask. These guys are experts at putting people to sleep. They have tranquilizers and sleeping pills and, for all I knew, laughing gas.

Then I started to get a bit nervous. I was in no shape to move or defend myself. What if this nutcase tried to hide in my room?

The ranting (and I don't mean the made-for-TV-commentary kind) continued for a while.

Incredibly, the nurses and orderlies defused the situation without a major catastrophe, and I would have bet on the catastrophe.

I'll bet he couldn't go #2, either.

While I still hadn't delivered the all-important #2, I got promoted out of the ICU into the surgery ward on the second day after surgery.

I felt good, mostly because I was still on heavy drugs. In fact, every time somebody would ask me something that I couldn't or didn't want to answer I'd chuckle and say, in my best imitation of a stoner in a *Harold & Kumar* movie, "Whadaya want? I'm on drugs, man."

It took maybe a day and a half for Barbara to gently tell me, "You can only use that for so long." That meant, of course, that I'd already overused it.

My wife, kids and sister were all there when it became time to move me. The mood was celebratory: I was well enough to get out of the ICU.

My family all grabbed my stuff—unread book, clothes, Sudoku puzzles, and the Hathaway Shirt ad—and started to walk me out of my room as an attendant pushed me on a gurney.

All of a sudden, the physical therapist strolled up and started asking me if she could give me an assessment test. I said, "Yes, but not right now. Can you wait until I'm in my new room?"

And then, at almost the same time, *The Good Doctor* appeared with a couple of residents in tow and started to give me some instructions. It then occurred to me that I hadn't yet thanked her for saving my life.

I began to fumble out a heart-felt "thank you," and that's when it happened, I pulled a "Boehner"[1] and started to bawl like a baby. I hadn't cried since I was maybe five years old. But the convergence of my family, the physical therapist, the nice nurse, the people in the hallway, and *The Good Doctor* was just too much for me. I started to cry. I sobbed. All the emotions and tensions and fears of the operation came tumbling out in a cascading stream of tears. I was unbelievably embarrassed. Thankfully, the attendant had the wits to quickly push me down the hall and away from the crowd.

I was on drugs, man.

Sometimes I'm asked "How big was the incision?" or "Where was the tumor?" or "Do you have a big scar?" Basically, they want a layman's understanding of how large the Blob was and, implicitly, was it really all that serious? Was I really in a lot of trouble? Is there something gooey or icky they can tell their friends about?

I confess that I usually don't know how to answer these questions very well. Here's some of the findings from the MRI as reported in a memo to *The Good Doctor*:

> There is a large extra-axial mass lesion along the left occipital parietal convexity measuring approximately 6.8 x 5.4 x 6.5 cm. There is probable extension of this tumor to involve the superior sagittal sinus posteriorly. Constellation of findings is most consistent with meningioma.

As best as I understand it, that description means that the mass was in the back, left-hand side of the brain and about 2.7 inches by 2.1 inches by 2.6 inches in size. The doctor also thought that the mass would also involve an important blood vessel running along the top of the brain.

If a guy asked I would say, "Go home and have your wife make a fist. It's about that large." If it's a lady, I'd ask them to make a fist and compare it to a profile of my head, which usually resulted in an impressive "Ohhhhh." But sometimes I got a confused or "Doubting Thomas" look. You could almost see the gears in their head trying to wrap their mind around the idea of something that large and finding it incredulous. I could almost see them thinking, "Nah, that can't be true!"

So, to the extent that a picture is worth a thousand words, here's a picture of the back of my head in the hospital just before I was leaving to go home. Yes, it does look like a zipper. And, as it turned out, a zipper would have saved us all a bit of trouble later on.

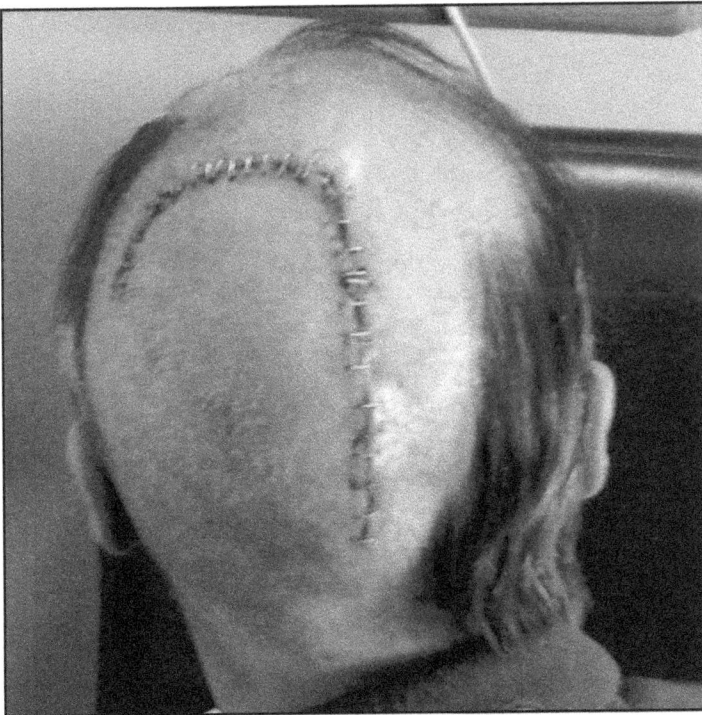

The picture of the back of my head that Barbara took the day I left the hospital

Well as it turns out, one of the prerequisites for leaving the hospital was going "#2." And while I hadn't eaten the stool softener pills like candy, I'd had more than my fair share. Nonetheless, the wheels of discharge were starting to slowly fall into place. I was taken down for an ultra-sound exam to see if I had any blood clots. I was taken for another MRI down in the low-lit bowels of the hospital. A counselor showed up and we talked about how I needed to enroll in occupational therapy, which is more about how to return to daily life than return to your job.

I also started to walk a little under the close supervision of a physical therapist. Strangely enough, I didn't walk as well as I had before the surgery. My right foot curled under a bit when I walked. How could that happen? Hadn't I been a runner since junior high school? Wasn't my balance pretty good? *The Good Doctor* hadn't operated on my foot. As it turned out, my ability to walk, like many other things I used to take for granted, had taken a few steps backwards. The over-arching answer was like a stock broker's warning: "past performance was no guarantee of future achievements" (especially when it comes to brain surgery).

This begged a question: What else wasn't working like it had prior to the operation? What was due to my continued heavy medicine prescriptions and what was an ongoing handicap? Was my vision better? Worse?

Maybe recovering from this operation was going to be a bit more difficult than I thought or hoped. Then again, I hadn't thought at all about the recovery period; all my attention was focused on the operation itself. I began to worry that this recovery business was going to be more of a marathon than a sprint.

But then it happened. The skies parted. The water dried up for Moses. And I went #2.

Yea!

3

Home (and Not) Alone

ACCORDING TO THE HOSPITAL'S RECORDS, I checked in on Thursday, October 28, and was discharged on Monday, November 1. Call it five days and four nights. Psychologically, however, it seemed much, much longer.

Home wasn't what I remembered. It wasn't that I was a *Stranger in a Strange Land*. It was that I was a "Stranger in a Familiar Land."

Well, what do I mean? I mean that the neighborhood hadn't changed, the house hadn't changed, the weather hadn't changed, but *I* had changed.

Under direction from the nurses, Barbara removed all the slippery "throw rugs" in the house, which would be like throwing a banana peel in front of Elmer Fudd (if you don't know who Elmer Fudd is, ask somebody who watches too many cartoons).

Our first floor really-good-imitation leather chair became my base of operations. It had a sturdy footstool on which I could stack papers, rehab materials and outdoorsy magazines.

Physically, I was still weak. I tired easily. And I wasn't yet sleeping more than maybe two to three hours a night.

In some ways I could better see what I couldn't see (if that makes any sense at all). My peripheral vision, which before the operation was non-existent, had turned into a smooshed Monet painting. More specifically, through the right side of my right eye I could see a cacophony of colors. The colors changed with the scenery, but I couldn't really see anything distinctly, like a waffle iron or a kitchen counter corner. While I was told that I hadn't lost any brain cells affecting my vision, we all knew that they had just been "squashed" and entangled with the tumor. We hoped that I might regain my peripheral vision over time. There was also a chance that I might not.

Away from the comfort of the hospital, I was forced to consider my future. It seemed uncertain, especially early on when I was still learning how to walk without curling my foot. Giving myself a status report, I told myself that on the positive side:

I was alive.
My family loved me and was unbelievably helpful.
Unlike many other brain tumor victims, I could talk, walk (well, sort of), and read.

On the negative side:

My eyesight was crappy.
I was physically and mentally fragile.
I was certain that my brain wasn't quite using all four cylinders.
And I had a bit of Blob left in me.

But by far the most immediate issue was to arrange a visit from my brother and parents.

As luck would have it, on the day of my operation my nephew was graduating from basic training in the Army. My dad, mother and brother had committed to seeing him at his graduation. In fact, prior to my operation date being moved up to the same day, I had planned to attend, too.

My wife (have I mentioned how perceptive she is?), was a bit worried about the entire Kerastas clan descending upon the hospital at once. As it was, we had my wife, our three children, my sister, my buddy Greg, and Pastor Jane in my hospital room for the MSU versus Iowa football game. If we'd added the rest of the Kerastas clan, well, we were worried about spontaneous combustion.

My sister and I knew that my parents would worry themselves to death until they came and saw for themselves that I was okay (or could at least fake being okay). So we scheduled my brother, father and mother to come visit us on the day after I was back home. And while I wasn't really up for chit-chat, I needed to put their minds at ease.

They booked a room at a nearby hotel, drove in from Michigan, and zipped over to the house that evening for a preliminary examination.

I hadn't slept well since coming home, and when I'm tired (or hungry), I tend to be a bit snippy. My job was to put my Mom's and Dad's minds at ease. I thought about this and resolved to be on my best behavior.

My folks and brother entered the house rather tentatively. This was a marked contrast to the shouting and hooting that usually ensues. (I think my Dad's booming "Hellos" are mostly due to his loss of hearing. If you go to their house while they're watching TV, you get the feeling that somebody is testing the upper limits of the TV set's volume.)

After the prelims were over, my eighty-six year old Dad marched over and plunked himself down on top of the brown imitation ottoman sectional in front of my chair. He was maybe two to three feet from me. He looked me straight in the eye with a fierceness that I hadn't seen for years and asked, "John, are you all right?"

Now, I mean, really. How do you answer something like that?

"Hell, I'm fit as a fiddle...a fiddle that got slammed in a car door."

"I can't sleep, I'm despondent about my crummy eyesight, and I'm pissed that I can't even walk right. Other than that, I'm just ducky."

"How the hell would I know? I'm on so many meds I don't know if I'm punched or stamped."

I probably choked out something like, "All things considered, not too bad." I think he then asked, "John, are they treating you all right?" I thought, who are "they?" My wife and my sister? No, they're ordering me around like a little kid, but I needed ordering. Did he mean the nurses? They weren't here; they were back at the hospital. So I sputtered and dribbled out something suitably inane like, "Dad, I'm pretty darn happy to be alive. I'm with the people I love. I'm in there slugging."

Of course, none of that meant squat, but I wanted to show him that I had a positive attitude and could talk. As I later found out, most people expected the worst—that you couldn't talk, that your IQ had sunk to new lows, or that you were handicapped in some strange and terrifying way. I don't blame them for those concerns.

Here's a great example, a note from a friend who'd heard about my tumor:

I'm glad to see you can type! My experience of brain surgery is largely confined to the movies where the patient awakes to a circle of concerned faces all waiting to see if he suddenly speaks in Urdu or thinks a carrot smells like a sausage and so on. But it seems you have woken up in fully functioning order!

Actually, I do have a brain operation story. My friend ____ had two seven-hour brain operations after suffering severe head injuries in a car accident. (He made a full recovery.) But when he awoke from the surgeries he had to spend several days in a delirium while the brain tissue healed. During this time he spoke only Spanish, a language he learned in South America while he was at school until the age of four and which he had completely forgotten in the intervening 35 years! Or so he thought.

The Brain. It really is the last frontier.

Given those perceptions, I tried to repeat my key messages to my worried and earnest father: "Dad, as far as brain tumors go, I'm pretty lucky. I can recover from this. My head does look like a mess. It might take a while. But I will recover."

It was good to repeat those messages because I needed to hear them too.

My Dad had heard what he needed to hear. He turned to my Mother and said, "We need to leave and let John rest." I stood up. I gave my Mom a hug. She got a little teary and my bear of a brother ushered them out of the house and into the car.

When they came back the next day, they seemed satisfied with what they found. I was given softball questions for which I offered up reassuring answers. I tried to take a mid-morning nap, dozed a little, and they were gone when I got up.

Our House (is a Very, Very, Very Fine House). It's also old. In 1988 we received a letter from a lady who claimed that she reckoned it turned 100 years old that year. Why did she think so? She claimed that her father had built the house in 1888. Her letter was full of tantalizing historical anecdotes. For instance, her letter went on to say that she remembered playing their piano in the parlor when they heard that Italy invaded Ethiopia. And, almost as an afterthought, she also mentioned that soon after Mussolini invaded Ethiopia, she and her family moved to China as missionaries. I thought, hmmm, a bad time to be moving to China given the impending Communist revolution and the Japanese invasion.

Thanks to her grandfather, we now had a comfortable old house full of high ceilings, hardwood floors and big windows. It also meant that while our house was old, drafty and creaky, it also had a certain amount of charm you won't find in a typical Midwest post-World War II suburb. A good visual reference would be Jimmy Stewart's house in the movie, *It's a Wonderful Life.*

In our house, you can also hear anybody moving around on the squeaky hardwood floors. So I tried to keep my middle-of-the-night sounds to a minimum. It also meant that any light sleeper would know if I was breaking one of the "Rules."

The Rules

Before I explain the rules, I guess I need to explain that my sister, the Greatest Sister in the World™, had volunteered to stay with me from the day I got home from the hospital until Thanksgiving. That was a significant sacrifice on her part because she had just started attending Southern Oregon University as part of her own continuing education effort.

By way of explanation, she's a Doctor of Oriental Medicine who sails the seven seas (yes, all seven) on a cruise ship healing rich patients who, oftentimes, are taking a gazillion pills. As she tells it, not knowing what all these pills do inhibits her ability to treat her patients. As a result, she decided to get some Western medical education so that her treatments would be even better.

To that end, she asked for time off from the cruise line to take the basic science courses she needed to pass to take even more relevant medical courses. When she learned of my plight, she decided to plea her "Leave of Absence" case with her professors, come to the Chicago area and proctor me during my early convalescence. She wasn't asked; she just said she'd do it and return to school in time for her final exams. Doing so was a big relief to Barbara who was concerned about me being home alone.

Now, that's a sister.

I should also tell you that she's not quite five feet tall and has reddish-brownish hair and freckles. She is a master at making up stories to tell young children around campfires. She spent over twenty years being intimately involved with the Appalachia Service Project (a terrific non-profit agency). And, along with my brother, she's one of my personal heroes.

Having said all that, at the beginning of my at-home recovery, Barbara and Nancy made sure one rule was clear: I wasn't supposed to go "walking around" without Barbara or Nancy there to make sure I didn't fall and injure myself. That meant no "getting out of a chair to go to the bathroom by myself," no "waltzing into the kitchen to make a sandwich by myself," and no "walking the dog by myself."

Easy, right? Wrong.

Here's why: Coming out of surgery, people are constantly telling you what you can't do, what you shouldn't do, and what you shouldn't even think about doing. It makes you feel inadequate, disempowered, and much less than you used to be. This all comes at a time when you yearn for reassurance that everything will be all right, that you will be able to work and earn a living, that you will be able to enjoy your old hobbies, that you'll be attractive to your wife, and that you won't be looked upon with pity.

The idea that you can't even go to the bathroom without a handler is humiliating. I mean, if I can't do that, what can I do?

This also gets at a puzzle of the recuperation process. According to everything I've read and heard, it's important to have a positive attitude during your recovery. Yet, at the same time, most of the feedback you get is negative, it's what you *can't* do.

I was also full of "Why me?" I had, and I suspect other victims have as well, a lot of pent-up anger about getting a brain tumor. Neither of my parents and none of my grandparents had a brain tumor. I went to church regularly, and contributed time and money to charity (never enough, though). I didn't cheat on my wife, drink to excess, or bet the kids' college education fund at the blackjack table. So why did I get the short stick? It wasn't fair. And as much as I tried to tell my ego to stop that unproductive, negative line of thinking, it was constantly lurking in the back of my mind trying to drag me into dangerously deep and dank psychological waters.

Now here was my conundrum: Nancy was the enforcer of the rules. Had anybody else—my Mom, Pastor Dean—been enforcing the rules, I would've been a bad patient, a sarcastic patient, a whiny patient.

But Nancy softly explained that my head was still quite fragile and the consequences of falling down were severe. Even I could read the neon signs between the lines that said "she hadn't come all the way to the Chicago area to see me throw away my life."

Said differently, I got the unspoken but unmistakable message that if I fell, cracked my head open, and died; Nancy and Barb would resurrect me and kill me all over again.

So I tried hard to obey the rules and not grumble...too loudly.

When I was in the hospital I had to manage three differing interest groups:

> The hospital staff
> My friends and family
> My ego

By far and away, my ego was the toughest to manage. If your ego is, at some level, based on your work performance, *not* being able to work eliminates an important part of the positive feedback you expect to receive.

If you buy into "look smart, feel smart, be smart," and then get a shock when you look into a mirror and see Gabby Hayes, you're probably not a happy camper. That's a good description of how I felt and looked (by the way, Gabby was a crusty and hairy yet likeable sidekick in a ton of cowboy films in the '30s and '40s).

If you love getting up early, jumping on your bike for 40 miles and then can't, you wonder if you'll be able to do so again.

And so, while *The Blob* physically injured my brain, it really wounded my pride and ego.

Under those conditions, every slight cuts deeper. The deepest cuts, the ones that really sting your ego, are often the comments made when somebody is trying to be nice to you or protect you. Not being "allowed" to walk by myself was one such deep cut. It was a rule made to be broken.

Breaking the Rules

There's something about *trying* to sleep that just makes you more awake. The more upset you get about it, the harder it is to do, much like golf. I'd lie in bed until I couldn't stand it anymore, and then ask Barb to escort me down to the first floor chair where I'd camp out. Since she's a night owl, she probably just fell into a deep sleep when this goofball of a husband would wake her up.

Once downstairs, the understanding was that I was to *stay in that chair* and call for assistance should I, say, need to visit the "loo." Was this embarrassing? Yes. Did I follow the rules? Well, about the third night, those dang stool softener pills kicked in...in high gear. That was a good thing, because I needed to start a more natural rhythm in that area.

It was about 3 a.m. and I was sitting on my faux leather brown chair in the living room when the urge suddenly struck me. So I used a stage whisper to call my sister who was sleeping in a second floor bedroom (the closest bedroom to my downstairs chair).

"Nannnncy," I hissed.

No response. My intestines started to roll and buckle.

"Nannnnnnnnncy," I sung out softly.

My lower abdomen started to gurgle ominously.

"Hey! Nancy," I said somewhat loudly.

Nothing.

"Nance."

I started to strain.

"Pance." She hated that childhood nickname.

Well here was my choice: Soil myself or break the rules. I broke the rules (you would, too!) and walked calmly and safely to the downstairs bathroom.

After a certain period of relief, I started to wonder. Hmmmm, should I flush the toilet? If I flush it and wake somebody up, they'll know that I broke the rules.

On one hand, if I slink back to my chair and don't flush, they would find a little surprise in the downstairs toilet which would be hard to explain. I started to discuss this little issue with myself. How did I do that, you ask? With some difficulty, I must say, but let me recap the conversation in Freudian terms:

ID: "Screw 'em you wimp, and go into the kitchen and make yourself some bacon and eggs."

Superego: It would be wrong to lie to your wonderful sister and lovely wife about all this."

Ego: "Are you guys nuts? I'm going to flush the toilet and fuggedaboutit."

And I did.

For the first two weeks home, I still couldn't sleep much. The first two weeks were murder, I'd get maybe an hour and a half, maybe two hours before waking up. I'd then lie there until I felt I could wake up Barb or Nancy to be escorted down to the first floor.

I was still on potent drugs and felt mentally slow. As I mentally wrestled with this problem, mostly at 3 a.m. in the morning, I remembered something about the "Mozart Effect" which found that listening to classical music was good for brain-damaged patients. "Well," I thought, "I'm brain-damaged. Shouldn't this be helpful for me?"

Did I do a lengthy investigation of the research? I think you know me well enough by now to know that I never let the facts get in the way of a good story.

I flipped through my thin collection of Mozart. I had some symphonies and some French horn concertos. A brief listen told me all I wanted to know: they were too fancy, too frilly, too jaunty. Maybe I would have embraced Mozart's *Requiem Mass in D minor*, but I didn't have it.

Later that day Nancy and I walked over to the library in search of the right music. I wanted dark, complex, funereal Russian and Slavic and German Music, something with gravitas. On a trip to the library we found two CDs that fit the bill: *Heavy Classix* and *Heavy Classix Vol. 2*. The picture on the CD said it all: a robust woman wearing Viking battle armor and wearing a metal hat sprouting stout horns. She looked as if she'd rather stomp you than say "have a nice day."

That was exactly what I was looking for (no, not the woman), CDs full of unromantic, murky and foreboding music from Wagner, Mussorgsky, Stravinsky, Holst, Borodin and Shostakovich.

That night after waking up with another two to three hours of sleep I sat in my chair on the first floor in the dark at three and four in the morning, listening and scowling. My dog, Louis, gave me a wide berth.

Smart dog.

One day I got the following email:

The gentleman below and I go back a long ways. He is opening a new division of a company and needs expert marketing help. I've recommended you. Please call and we can discuss.

An old boss of mine had recommended me for a position at a newly formed division of a larger firm. Since I was technically unemployed (my two key clients had both been bought or were being bought by larger companies), this was manna from heaven.

Then I stopped and thought for a minute:

I can't drive and the HQ of the office is 20 miles away.

My head is full of sutures the size of railroad ties.

Half my head is shaved and the hair on the other half is rather long.

My wife and sister don't even like me walking by myself just yet.

They say that you never have a second chance to make a good first impression, and even I could guess what kind of a first impression I would make. I called my old boss back, thanked him, but declined the opportunity.

For those of you keeping score at home, I had been a free-lance marketer ever since my previous company was bought out from underneath me. And, since the economy was still in the toilet, the idea of a full-time job falling into my lap was something akin to experiencing Nirvana, discovering King Tut's tomb and becoming self-actualized all rolled up into one.

Having to admit to a former boss, whom I greatly admired, that I was incapable of tackling that opportunity was like puncturing my little balloon of an ego with a needle and watching it whizz around the room until it ran out of gas and lay limp on the floor.

I felt lower than whale shit.

Barbara was back at her taxing job at the ad agency and sent the following email to friends and family:

Good morning!

I realized yesterday that I probably needed to send a new status on John—given that he was still in the ICU the last time. Yikes—sorry about that!

The fact is John is home and doing really, really well. He was moved to a regular room at the hospital on Friday afternoon, less than 24 hours after surgery, and was eating regular food and taking short walks that afternoon. At the moment, he is experiencing some deficit in his right peripheral vision. They will continue to monitor this and hope it will improve as John recovers. He came home on Monday and is taking pretty long walks already. This morning, he got up, made breakfast for himself and is attempting today's Sudoku puzzle.

Not bad considering he was in surgery one week ago.

Thank you all for the kind thoughts along this journey.

Barb and John

This is when we learned who our real friends were; real friends bring you food when you are too tired or too sick to do it yourself.

It's also when I learned that American comfort food is chili. I used to think that there are three kinds of chili: mild, medium and hot. Au contraire! Chili comes in colors and feet. If you are from the Midwest you know that you can have no feet (vegetarian), two feet (chicken and turkey), or four feet (beef, pork and hamster). On the color scale, chili comes in white, brown, green, red and possibly some colors I forgot. I'm still trying to pry the brown chili recipe out of Greg wife's Donna, but I think her secret ingredient is chocolate.

Food was also delivered in bulk. Barbara's office ordered up a gazillion helpings of food to be delivered to the house.

But just as you can't out-gift the Japanese[3], you can't out-feed the Methodists. Methodists came in droves. They came as individuals. They came as teams. They brought homemade salads, breakfast breads, appetizers, desserts, coffee cakes, casseroles, and, of course, more desserts.

Now I'm going to get into dangerous territory and admit that this "you can't out-feed" the Methodists is somewhat of a sectarian statement. I readily confess that I've seen terrific spreads put out by the Shinto's and Buddhists in Japan. I've eaten an amazing home-cooked Indian meal that took days to prepare. I've feasted on Thai food beyond any reasonable calorie count. And I've certainly had lots of Catholic meals as well as various Protestant buffets.

But pound-for-pound, I don't think you can "out-feed" the Methodists (although I'm a bit worried about the Southern Baptists).

And as much as I love gourmet food from a gourmet store, there is something supremely comforting about unrequested homemade food that you just can't buy off the shelf.

Methodist hospitality extended, if you can believe it, beyond food. When I needed watching because Nancy had to take time off for a funeral, the irrepressibly positive Pastor Jane or my Appalachia Service Project ("ASP") partner in teen herding and ditch digging, Mary, would come and keep me company (i.e. watch me like a hawk) until Barbara could get home.

This was, of course, somewhat of a double-edged sword, as I now have no moral high ground from which to turn down any request of Pastor Jane's (which means that I'm going to be schlepping down to Appalachia on high school ASP trips when I'm 80 years old).

At this point in my recovery, I just looked goofy. Part of my head was shaved for the operation but starting to make a comeback. Other patches of hair were oddly long, having not been cut for weeks. And then I also had a mangy beard germinating in several directions at once. My head looked like a poorly built tri-level house from the 1970s.

Nancy and I agreed that I needed to get a haircut to at least get all the hair at the same level.

So one cold and unfriendly November day we hoofed it down to Jerry's barber shop about a half mile from our house. Jerry's is the kind of barber shop that all guys are immediately comfortable in: linoleum floors, lots of sports and car magazines, and a cheap radio tuned onto an oldies station. You can walk in wearing shorts and a tee shirt, a sport coat and matching pants, or a sweat shirt and sweat pants, nobody cares.

It's the kind of place where there's a coat rack that nobody uses.

Jerry's is run by a mob of women with vaguely Middle Eastern accents that I could never identify: Armenian? Turkish? Lebanese? Who knew? They cut kid hair, teenage hair, and old man hair.

Nancy and I shuffled in from the cold November weather and plopped ourselves down in a couple of chairs. The dark-haired proprietress soon motioned to an empty sea. So I ambled over and settled in. She then talked to one of the female barbers and asked her to cut my hair.

The designated barber approached cautiously and gave my sorry-looking head with railroad-sized stitches a good long look. She then shook her head with a nod of conviction and walked away.

There was then a brief but animated discussion in their language, which, I assumed, went something like this:

"Whatsa matta with you?"

"Whatsa matta with me? Have you looked at his head?"

"He's a customer! A paying customer!"

"His head looks like Mom's moussaka when we left it out for a week during vacation."

"You're dating Yanni and all of a sudden you're picky?"

"I've seen diseased goats I'd rather touch!"

"Wimp!"

"And his zits are ugly."

"Okay, I'll cut his hair and show you how a real woman treats a customer."

And she did. Slowly, gently, and precisely she trimmed the old growth, new growth, and my mangy beard. Afterwards I looked, well, about as good as I could look. She charged maybe $20 and I gave her a $10 tip. And, while she probably knows it, she also has a customer for life.

One of the several things I did absolutely wrong prior to my first surgery was not tell *all* my friends. In fact, I really only told a few, very close friends. Why didn't I? I was under some strange delusion that if "work" friends found out, maybe they wouldn't want me to work on their projects. I could imagine the following conversation back at HQ:

"Fred, who do you want to help out on the Ontario projects?"

"I was thinking of asking Kerastas."

"I remember him. What's he been doing?"

"Oh, he's been recovering from a brain tumor operation the last several months."

"Explain this to me and use simple words because I don't understand this idea at all."

At the same time, I felt somehow embarrassed to admit to having a brain tumor. Why was this embarrassing? I'm not really sure, but it made me feel "less," and I wasn't emotionally ready to admit that I was certainly different and probably something less than what I was.

But I was feeling guilty about not telling guys that I'd worked with for years. So after the operation I finally sent Barbara's original email about my brain tumor to one of my good work friends as well as her follow-up email:

> Dear ____,
>
> I thought you should know that I've had a bit of a health challenge (see attached). Please give my best to ____.
> John

Well, he read the first email, thought I was soon having the operation and promptly enlisted his entire family to put me on their prayer list. He then reread the email and sent me the following:

> You stinker. When I called you a few minutes ago it was from the BB (*i.e., BlackBerry*) and I understood the surgery to be this Thursday, but now reading the whole email on my computer, I see it was last Thursday. So I missed the whole thing and now you're home and recovering.

I felt awful. I had misled a good friend and better person. But wait! It gets worse. I sent the following email to an old boss of mine which included, as an attachment, Barbara's original announcement email:

> Dear ____,
>
> I have wanted to apologize for my lack of contributions to the Ontario projects last year. I now somewhat recently better understand why this - see attached (attached was Barbara's first note explaining that I had a tumor and would be undergoing surgery).
> All the best,
> John

As I reread this, I cringe. I was trying to be nonchalant and put this tumor business behind me. His email back to me was honest and accurate and, rightfully so, it stung.

> Not an issue. I wish I had known earlier about this—I would have kept you in my prayers.
> It sounds like things are going well. I'm not sure that sarcasm in the ICU is a good idea - but you probably can't help yourself.
> You need flowers or beer?"

Actually, I needed whiskey and didn't deserve the good stuff. I just relived my previous errors on "How not to tell somebody." What did I learn from all this? I think I learned that a health issue isn't something to be hidden or be embarrassed about. If they are really your friends, they want to know at the earliest moment. If they aren't your friends, don't worry about what they think.

I decided to win Dr. Rosseau's "Patient of the Month" award. Now I wasn't sure she was even thinking of creating such an award, but I told Nancy that our goal was for me to be so healthy at the six-week mark, our first big review, that she would have to create the award and give it to our family as a total effort, sort of like the Oscar for the "Best Picture" when everybody comes up on stage.

Being overly goal oriented, I created three goals for myself:

Regain normal physical activity, like walking,
Take advantage of my sister's doctorial skills (i.e., acupuncture) to accelerate my healing,
Regain normal vision and cognitive skills.

In terms of physical activity, *The Good Doctor* laid down the law: she wanted me to be walking one and a half miles a day by our appointment at the six-week mark, December 2.

Finally, here was something I could do to help the healing process. I jumped on it like a hobo on a ham sandwich.

I started measuring the walking distance to local landmarks: the library, the Starbucks, and the local grocery stores. In true Kerastas overkill fashion, each day Nancy, Louis and I would take at least two walks (and sometimes three).

Since I wanted to prove that I was delivering on my promise, I kept a daily log of where we walked to, and how far we went. I kept stats on our daily mileage and how that affected our overall cumulative average. And, hooray, I exceeded the Doctor's prescribed goal of 1½ miles a day in the first day.

Yes, I was anal about it.

When I got to a day when we logged over 6 miles, I called *The Good Doctor's* patient assistant and asked them if there was any benefit in going for seven, eight, or nine miles a day? At first she seemed a bit confused by the question. After a bit of explaining, she assured me that three miles a day was plenty, and that I should spend my time doing other things, like working on my occupational rehab activities.

What occupational rehab activities? Well, the nice rehab specialist gave me a couple of tests on the first day we met. One of the first tests was a hand-administered eye exam, which was illuminating, if nothing else.

To my surprise, I still had substantial blindness. The upper right-hand quarter of my right eye was almost totally blind. How did this happen? I thought the operation was supposed to fix all this. Or did I just *hope* it would fix all this?

More disturbing at the time, however, was a small wedge of blindness in the upper left-hand corner of my left eye. I had this vague memory of a hospital therapist telling me that you can drive if you are blind in one eye, but you can't if you have even a smidgeon of blindness in the other eye, too.

In *my* opinion I only had a "smidge" of blindness in my left eye, which was two letters less than a "smidgeon," and no reason why I shouldn't be able to drive.

The idea that I wouldn't be able to drive was a bit unnerving on every front I could imagine:

I hated asking for a ride to, well, anywhere before I got my driver's license. Was I going to have to relive those days? "Gee, Barbara, could you please drive me over to Meier's Tavern so I could have a shot and a beer with the guys?"

Would I be demoted to pre-sixteen-year-old status by my wife?

My Dad worked at the Ford Motor Company for 35 years or so and made it very clear that we would have to "pry his cold dead hands from his car keys." Would I lose my rights as an adult American to drive without a fight?

How could I get to work if I couldn't drive?

More importantly, who would hire me if I couldn't drive?

And lastly, would I never again be a designated driver (well, maybe it wasn't all bad)?

I also wanted to regain my physical strength and reflexes (and flush out the anesthetic from the operation) ASAP. So after hearing this rather sobering news about my inadequacies, we pulled out our secret weapon, Nancy.

Nancy put together an acupuncture program designed to accelerate my recovery. For some of you, including Western doctors, the thought of acupuncture for a patient who just had brain surgery would be a bit crazy. I still run into many folks who assume that acupuncture is voodoo science, i.e. unproven and possibly dangerous practices for new-age, airy-fairy types grasping at straws. I had a doctor physically gasp, stretch her eyebrows to the ceiling and put her hands on both sides of her cheeks when I told her that I had acupuncture after brain surgery.

My first impressions of acupuncture were not all that dissimilar. But a few years ago, after a day spent helping my parents move out of their old house, my left knee locked up on me. It wasn't going to bend: "not no way, not no how."[2] I was sure I'd need somebody to haul me down to the hospital. But Nancy told me that she might be able to fix it with acupuncture. So I laid down on my Mom's impossibly comfortable rust-orange sofa and let Nancy stick me with a slew of acupuncture needles. The next day, my leg was absolutely normal. I've been a convert ever since.

So when she said she could help my recovery I said, "Sounds good to me." She started small. My first acupuncture treatment consisted of three needles, with none in the head. On most nights, just before bedtime, Nancy and I would head up into a spare bedroom where she would give me an acupuncture treatment. This consisted of inserting an increasing number of needles into classic acupuncture areas to help flush out the anesthetic, increase blood flow to my brain, and tackle those sneaky Shingles, among other things.

Oh, I forgot to mention them. It seems like Shingles (sort of an older and nastier brother of chicken pox) hides in your nerve endings and waits until you've had a bit of bad health and then—Wham!—reappears like crabgrass in your lawn. (Yes, that does sound creepy; and no, I don't know exactly where it hides in your nerve endings. I have enough trouble finding my house key.)

By November 23, that last day she stayed with us and gave me a treatment, I remember her telling me that she used over 100 needles in a treatment, which I think made me look like a "Hellraiser"[4] movie poster (actually, I'm just imagining that, she never gave me a mirror during my treatments).

Just before Thanksgiving, my wound looked great. I felt great. I was convinced that I was a shoo-in for that *Patient of the Month* award, and I attributed a great deal of the credit to my superb Western and Eastern doctor teams.

We drove to the Detroit area for Thanksgiving to visit with relatives on both sides of the family. Nancy would then return to Oregon for her final exam in anatomy and biology.

At that time, I felt that I had accepted my eyesight problem and was ready to tackle life anew. I felt physically strong. I felt in control. I felt I was moving rapidly in the right direction.

Little did I know that in less than a week, I would be back in the hospital and the back of my head would look worse than a diseased goat...a lot worse.

4

I'll Be Home for Christmas (I Hope)

THE THANKSGIVING HOLIDAY WAS REJUVENATING. We saw a variety of relatives that we hadn't seen since my operation. In almost every case I felt like they expected the worst: that I drooled, slurred my words or wouldn't be able to carry on a normal conversation. As I told them about the operation, showed my fierce scars and recounted my rehab regimen, I felt proud. I had taken the *Blob's* best blow and lived to tell about it. I was convinced that my prior good health, healthy eating and anal attention to walking would let me return to normal life in record time. I was going to win the *Patient of the Month* award hands down.

When we returned to the Chicago area and picked up Louis from the kennel, the weather had gone from Indian summer to Chicago Winter. Temperatures dipped under 32°. The wind gusted to 40 mph. And for the first time, snow fell. At the time we felt pretty smug. By historical standards, the Tuesday, November 29th flurries were late, as the first snow usually hits us around November 5th. Nonetheless, the change in weather was also a reminder that the warm and easy days of our beautiful, extended "Indian Summer" were over. It was now time to hunker down for tougher times, for short days and long dark nights, for the cold, dark days of winter up north.

My head also told me that my easy days were over, literally. On the Monday morning after Thanksgiving, just as I started to pick out my clothes for the day, Barbara picked up my pillow case and showed it to me. It was spattered with horrible-looking green and yellow pus.

She asked me to sit down and let her have a look at the back of my head. It looked worse.

Nancy's ministrations hadn't been stopped for a week, and my head started leaking like a burst water pipe. I didn't know how bad it was, but I knew it wasn't good news. Barb was being stoic, which just made me more nervous.

Unlike most burst pipes, we couldn't really tell where the leak was coming from: was it the skin? The skull? Something deeper and more ominous? The possibilities seemed to be of two varieties, bad and worse.

We already had an appointment set up for Tuesday afternoon with *The Good Doctor* and we went to see her as a whirlwind of fears swirled through our thoughts.

At first she wasn't as concerned (she's seen a lot of bad heads). But after telling her that this was a significant turn for the worse, she organized an appointment with an infectious disease specialist down at the Advocate Illinois Masonic hospital in the city.

This meant that I could take the "El" train (the train that ran on the electric tracks) down to the hospital by myself, Barbara could go to work and I could tell her what the doctor said after she got home.

The Masonic Hospital is in a trendy part of town at the corner of Wellington and Sheffield in Chicago. Great-looking rehabbed brownstones populate most every street in the area. Everywhere I looked, I saw young mothers pushing babies in spiffy European strollers that probably cost more than my first car (and since my first car was a Pinto, this could have very well been true).

The infectious disease doctor's office was on an upper floor of an office building adjoining the hospital. It had a great view of the surrounding area which, in spite of the crappy weather, still looked awfully nice. Her office was calming and, unlike the ophthalmologist's office, anything but antiseptic. She had modern art hanging on walls, interesting scents wafting through the air and contemporary furniture to sit on. Her office reeked of "modernity" and "success."

As *The Good Doctor* had snuck me onto her busy schedule as a favor, she was all business. Shortly after being shown to an examination room, she strode in the office, asked me a few basic questions and then took a good, long look at the back of my head. She then sat down in front of me, stared me straight in the eyes and said, "I want you to go to the hospital, did you pack a bag?"

It's time for a spot quiz: when she said "Go to the hospital, did you pack a bag?" she meant (pick one):

A. "You realize how serious this is, right?"
B. "Don't pass go and don't collect $200."
C. "You're in big trouble."
D. All of the above

If you picked "D," you're right.

I now had to make an interesting phone call to Barbara (have I said how composed she is when receiving bad news?). I called Barbara from the downstairs lobby, and said something like, "Here's a surprise, the infectious disease doctor doesn't like puss and goo dripping out of the back of my head. She wants me to go to straight the hospital." (By now I think you know that I don't really sugar coat things. If this is a surprise, go back and reread the Chapter 2 section on "How Not to Tell Everybody.")

I told her that I could take the "El" up to the Evanston Central Street station adjacent to the hospital, but she wouldn't hear of it. She made it clear that she was going to drive to the Masonic Hospital, take me home to pack a bag, and then we would meet *The Good Doctor* at the hospital.

As I waited in the minimally furnished first-floor lobby I watched busy doctors purposely stride in and out of the office building. I saw cabbies zoom by the medical office building in search of fares. They all seemed quite normal, busy, occupied.

Seconds ticked by. I thought about my head, my wound and what caused it. How bad could it be, I wondered? And the thought hit me, pretty bad. If the infection breached the brain's protective, err, layer (Tissue? Inner wall? Moat?), this would not end well. Would I become "Old Yeller"[1] with some disastrous brain disease chained to a stake in the back yard? Would I drool a lot? Foam at the mouth? Would they send Eric out with a shotgun to "do the right thing?"

Minutes ticked by. I was not in a happy place (No, not the vestibule of the office building, I meant "mentally").

After what seemed like an eon, but was probably closer to 20 minutes, Barbara pulled up in front of the building. I hopped into our SUV and she started to drive us north. We decided to go home to get me some PJ's before checking into the hospital. (You might be surprised to learn that I was not a big fan of the hospital's gowns. They only came in one color and clashed with my Mediterranean skin.)

Time for another pop quiz: at the same time I was being told to go to the hospital I believe that *The Good Doctor* was:

A. In surgery at a hospital far from the Evanston NorthShore Hospital.
B. Working out for another marathon.
C. Boarding a plane for a much deserved vacation in the South Pacific.
D. Preparing for her trip to Libya where she was scheduled to deliver a speech on (something to do with) brain surgery to (some important) committee of the Organization of African States.

If you picked "D," you're either clairvoyant or realize that "D" is always the right answer in my quizzes. (And, "yes," December 2010 was an interesting/fortuitous time to visit Libya.)

We met *The Good Doctor* on the first floor of the hospital and she pulled us into what seemed like a mailroom behind the welcome desk. She then told the local staff that she needed the space for a meeting and they left. As far as I can tell, *The Good Doctor* has that effect on everyone. As we sat in the mailroom, she explained that she was handing me off into the capable hands of a terrific infectious disease doctor while she caught a plane to Libya. At that moment, things didn't feel right. Here was the neurosurgeon that, in my opinion, saved my life and brain, and she was not only leaving the country, she was leaving the continent.

A few minutes later, we were checking into a room on 4th floor that faced east and, as a result, didn't give us a view of the Baha'i Temple which seemed like another bad sign. The infectious disease doctor explained that by sticking an IV in me he could give me antibiotics that were eleven times stronger than any pills they could give me. And he expected that after a couple of days (three at the most) I would have this pesky infection under control and get to go home. I thought that three days wouldn't be so bad. Louis will hardly miss me.

The Bottom 10%

Not surprisingly, I knew most of the nurses in the ward. I was a bit surprised, though, that they were still talking to me. In fact I slide a little too easily into my role as patient. I knew when to order food, when I'd get my vitals checked and what I should and shouldn't do. Since, at first, all I had to do was sit there and have my IV changed every couple of hours or so, I was a good patient and, after the first day, pretty bored. So I asked for a laptop to continue to work on my online cognitive rehab lessons.

Against all odds, they wheeled one of the floor's spiffy mobile laptops into my room. When Nancy was still in town, she had taken me to an outpatient rehab clinic to begin my cognitive rehab. I wasn't sure that I needed "cognitive" rehab, but wanted to be a good patient and play along. During my initial assessment session, my therapist had signed me up for an account with Lumosity, an online brain exercise site. It was surprisingly good. The online exercises all looked and felt like video games, only these games worked on different aspects of your braininess: your speed of decision making, your ability to pay attention, your short-term memory (or lack thereof), your problem solving (i.e. math) ability and your mental flexibility skills (i.e. multi-tasking, vocabulary and mental discipline).

"This is great!" I thought as I lingered over a cup of coffee from my morning's breakfast. I wheeled my IV stand over to a chair by the computer and started to go through the program they'd set up for me.

The first program was a short-term memory exercise. Hmmmm, this seemed simple. All I had to do was remember the shape of the last object (triangle, square, circle, etc.) I saw on the screen and push a button that indicated that the new object which appeared on the screen was the same or different from the last one. I first saw a purple square.

Somebody walked by and said "hi." Then, all of a sudden, something new was on the screen, a blue circle. Now was the first object a blue circle?

I thought. I squirmed. I tried to conjure up a mental picture…but, nothing conjured. Was it a blue circle? Ummm, no…I mean, yes…wait-a-minute, I don't think so. I pushed the "different" button. Aha! I was right.

A new object appeared, a yellow triangle. I stared out the window, dang, I can't see the Baha'i Temple. Oh, yeah, what did I just see? It must have been, err, the purple square.

"Buzz," a cranky sound emanated from the program, wrong!

I continued at this speedy pace through all five exercises

Every day I went through all the recommended exercises pre-programmed by my therapist. About the third day, I noticed this nifty little tab in the Lumosity program entitled "Your Profile." This tab gave you a status report of your mental performance in all five areas compared to everybody else on the site that were within five years of your age (millions have signed up).

I checked out my performance: on every mental performance indicator I was in the bottom 10th percentile. Said differently, on every measure 90% of my age-group peers made quicker decisions, paid better attention, remembered more, were better at problem solving and were more mentally flexible than me.

Shit.

But wait, it gets worse! This site is predominantly used for folks who *need* to work on their cognitive skills. So compared to the general public in my near-geezer age bracket, I was probably doing even worse.

For somebody who proudly graduated from Michigan State University and was grappling with an ominous head infection, this was like throwing an anchor to a drowning sailor. If this news got out to anybody who I worked with, I was dead meat. The first start-up I worked at was filled with super high-IQ types: MBAs from Stanford and University of Chicago, and PhDs. from Northwestern University. If you weren't "smart" nobody wanted to talk to you, let alone work with you.

Now if you weren't in the business world I worked in, you might think that business meetings were all about solving important problems, like analyzing supply chain bottlenecks and assessing new technology opportunities.

No way! I learned early in my career, that the first agenda item of most meetings was primarily about establishing who was the "smartest guy in the room"[2] and, only secondarily about how to move the business ahead. For example, if you presented a strategy document, everybody in the room would jump on you like a defensive lineman on a fumbled football to demonstrate that *they* were smarter and had better ideas. Why?

A. To support needy egos.
B. To make themselves feel mucho better by verbally berating others.
C. To leverage the idea that the *smartest guy* should also have the highest position and, ergo, be paid the most.
D. All of the above.

As usual, the answer is "D."

Needless to say, this adroit management and team-building technique was also known as "the last man standing" method of determining key strategic direction for many of the top tier businesses in the country. Enron is a great example of how this astute business process smartly impacts shareholder value.

Given my Lumosity scores, though, I would be hard-pressed to convince anyone in the room that I was the "smartest guy in the room" or even one of the smartest guys in the room or even deserved to be in the room.

In the spirit of "make lemonade out of lemons," I decided that I could reposition myself against that elitist and uber-capitalistic point-of-view by repositioning myself as the "dumbest guy in the room." As the guy who would be "at one" with the common man. As the guy who would never "over-think" anything. As the guy who went to Michigan State, not Stanford or University of Chicago or Northwestern. Hey, since I was in the lowest 10th percentile, who in the room would argue with me?

I imagined myself in some big, important cross-functional meeting and asserting "I'm the dumbest guy in the room and even I know that idea stinks!" This could be a whole new opportunity in consumer segmentation, *The Bottom 10%*. I could hire myself out and see if my fellow low-IQ types would understand a new product concept, figure out how to install a new software application or be able to pronounce a multi-syllable brand name.

I talked to a buddy of mine who suggested that us *Bottom 10%*ers could reposition ourselves as the "anti" or mirror image of MENSA by establishing ASNEM[3]: the American Society for Numbskulls and Everyday Morons.

But here was my conundrum: should I tell Barbara about my test scores? (Did I say how smart she is?) On one hand, she would be sympathetic. On the other hand, I would feel pathetic.

I decided not to. My ego was also mired in the *Bottom 10%*.

For the next several days, from a medical and emotional perspective, I felt like I was treading water. There was nothing I could personally do other than wait and see if the high-powered antibiotics dripping in through the IV worked their magic.

While waiting, the weather continued to worsen and become a real

Chicago-style winter. The wind blew, the temperature dropped, and folks would stagger into the hospital draped in all manner of winter gear: scarves, wellies, full-length down coats and arctic-tested gloves.

In contrast, our ward was rather toasty and most of us wore little more than the regulation hospital gowns. I had brought some pajama bottoms given my Midwestern modesty and interest in avoiding flashing anybody.

Every morning, one of the residents would come by my bed to check out my wound. They'd have a look, stymie a wince, and say something like, "This isn't progressing the way we'd like it to".

This is where holding your tongue is a virtue. In my experience you never get better medical attention with sarcastic or even caustic remarks, no matter how good it'll make *you* feel. I remember thinking, however:

"Are you feeling okay? When you were looking at my wound it sounded like you were starting to retch."

"The 'airsick' bags are on my nightstand."

"Is that strained look on your face due to lack of fiber in your diet?"

After a few days the Head of Neurosurgery dropped by my room. He introduced himself and said (here's the Cliff notes version) if I didn't turn around by the following morning they would have to assume that the skin on my scalp was infected. In that case, they'd need to "clean up" the wound and cut away the infected parts.

This would entail putting me in "twilight," not a full anesthetic knock-out, but something that would allow them to do some cutting and scraping. If that didn't work, they'd assume that the skull was infected. In which case, they'd need to cut out the infected bone.

Yipes! Hide the Radial Arm Saw! (Even if it did have Laser-Trac)

While I was worried, the worst part of this was calling and telling my folks about the impending "scraping." As I saw it, my job was to make them aware of the operation and make sure that they weren't in any way spooked. Since *I* was a bit spooked, this wasn't going to be as easy as it should have been.

So I called them and we had a little discussion that might have gone like this:

"Hi Mom! Hi Dad!"

"Hello, John. How are you?"

"Well, that's why I'm calling."

"Yesssss?"

"It seems like this darn infection just isn't going away like it should. So the doctor is going to perform a little procedure where he's going to cut away the infected skin."

"Son, are you going into the operating room?"

"Yes, but they didn't even ask me for a deposit on the room, so it's going to be quick."

"Isn't *The Good Doctor* out of the country? Who is going to do the operation?"

"Well, that's the good thing. Actually, I didn't mean it that way. I mean that the 'Head of Neurosurgery' is going to fill in for her, so I'm in very good hands."

"Well, you know we worry..."

"Aww, there's nothing to worry about. We have *The Good Doctor's* boss and he'll do a great job," I fibbed. (Now that came out wrong, too. I fibbed about not having anything to worry about, not about having any qualms about the Head of Neurosurgery).

"What if that doesn't work?" asked my father.

"No worries. This is a 'lay down' (in poker), a 'gimmie' (in golf), a 'Slam Dunk' (in basketball)." I stopped because I ran out of clichés.

I heard a sniffle from my Mom.

"Now, Mom" I said gently. Don't worry. Everything will be 'okay.' We'll give you a call after it's done with the good news."

On the day of the operation, they started me on a second IV just before wheeling me down to the main event. I was awake when we arrived in the operating room, which isn't particularly calming. Shortly, however, they turned up the juice and I drifted off.

I wasn't supposed to be awake during this procedure, but I remember starting to wake up and feeling the Head of Neurosurgery put in some stitches. I said something encouraging and cheery like "Hey! That hurts!" I suspect the anesthesiologist then ramped up the drugs because I fell back into "La-la" land awfully quickly.

After I woke up from the minor "clean-up" operation, one of the very competent nurses zipped into my room and told me about the pain medicine options. And when I say "zipped," I really mean it. She was a thin, high-energy marathoner who seemed to be auditioning for a part in a perpetual motion machine. And since I was auditioning for the part of a door stop, we were ripe fodder for a "compare and contrast" essay question.

In general, I don't like to take anesthetic unless I really need it. For example, when it comes to drilling and filling a cavity, I generally decline pain medicine. Now when I say this, most folks look at me with a quizzical, questioning, scrunched up face, "why not?" The simple answer is that I hate the woozy feeling that you get from anesthetics.

The more complex truth was that, in this case, I also didn't want to be any "slower" (mentally) than I already was. That *Bottom 10%* rating was kinda eating at me.

I also started remembering all those stories about regular guys who went into the hospital, had a few post-surgery pains, got buckets of pain pills, got hooked on the pain pills, and ended up dying while trying to rob Fort Knox so they could buy even more pain pills. Well sir, I wasn't going to be one of those guys!

So I declined everything but the absolute minimums and tried to go about my business of healing and making sure I didn't have to have a piece of my skull removed. The idea of having any part of my skull permanently removed spooked me. It just seemed like a major operation and one where things could easily go wrong. What if the surgeon sneezed while sawing through my skull, would I lose the use of left arm? My high school memories? My golf swing? Actually, none of those would be a great loss because my left arm can barely hold a baseball mitt let alone dribble a basketball, my high school memories are as embarrassing as everybody else's, and my golf game has a permanent duck hook (especially my drives).

If I did get a large piece of skull removed, would I wind up being one of those guys who always sets off the security alarm in the airport because of a steel plate in their head? If I wandered onto a construction site and was offered a hard hat would I just say "no thanks, I have a custom job that's embedded."

On the other hand, without a major portion of my skull, I could tell everybody I was "a few bricks shy of a load" and not be stretching the truth.

After the operation we waited for some evidence that the procedure worked. Every day a resident would come, examine my newly trimmed scalp and say something like "I don't like what I see."

Wait-a-minute! You know what happened to me? I was scalped! Isn't that scary? According to Wikipedia, "scalping is the act of removing another person's scalp or a portion of their scalp, either from a dead body or from a living person."

I've looked at the Head of Neurosurgery with a suspicious eye ever since.

All sorts of people visit you in the hospital. My buddy, Greg, was great at coming by and watching a football game or just hanging out. My grown-up children would come and sit with me, which was terrific.

In spite of my protestations, Barbara would come over every night after a full day's work, and walking the dog, to sit with me until she'd start nodding off.

And, once again, the Methodists came in droves. ASP buddies came, joked and told ASP stories. Pastor Jane strolled on over, literally, as her house was a block away from the hospital. She's the rare person who can talk to a three year old, a third-grader and a thirty three year old, and they all think she's cool. An infectious giggler and prankster, she talked about having a house full of high schoolers (yes, she's also fearless) over to the parsonage for a "secret Santa" gift exchange.

Pastor Dean, the senior pastor, also came by and checked on me, which was unnecessary but highly appreciated. And since we are the same age and both grew up in Michigan, we have a lot in common and a pretty similar sense of humor. But, since he's a Wolverine and I'm a Spartan, we have tribal differences that will always be the "elephant in the room" of our relationship. Tribal allegiances notwithstanding, he has this great laugh that comes from his belly and lights up his eyes. If he ever gets out of the church business and grew a beard, he'd make a great Santa Claus.

Our minister of pastoral care, Bob Keller, however, was a serious guy with a serious job, especially since many of the folks he visits are on the downhill slide. When he strides into your hospital room, you can just sense his gravitas. He appeared to be in his late seventies, gaunt and with just enough white hair to keep his head from being sunburned during short walks.

He's not the kind of guy, though, to avoid asking the tough questions, the disturbing questions, the questions that really sick patients often need to have asked.

In our church, he had a terrific reputation for a sincere, thoughtful and no-nonsense approach to these subjects. I, however, was searching for any excuse to envelope myself in the darkness of denial. So I grasped for any dumb joke or silly pun to help me avoid the seriousness of my situation. As you can imagine, this meeting was doomed from the get go.

The first question he asked me was something like, "how do you feel?" In my best stoner imitation, I think I answered, "I feel great, I'm on heavy drugs, man."

His forehead wrinkled. He looked somewhat shocked and said, "Is that supposed to be funny?"

He then asked me about a will, and I talked about visiting Jim Morrison's grave and how cool that seemed, but settling on the idea of being cremated with half the ashes being cast around the MSU Marching Band practice field and the other half being thrown into the wind on Mount Fuji.

He seemed like he wanted to ask a question, but thought better about it.

I then said something like I had a "Living Will" and wanted my family to pull the plug when I couldn't salivate at the thought of a Kuma burger, because whenever that happened, I was truly beyond hope.

This time he just stared at me.

I went on to say that I left all my worldly possessions to Barbara so that, when I was gone, she could take our hard-earned savings, find herself a good-looking gigolo, and enjoy herself.

That did it. He was ready to skedaddle. I'm not sure if he thought that I was either beyond hope or just plain hopeless. He offered to pray with me and left.

I think my decision not to tell him about the Baha'i temple was a good one.

I remember my youngest daughter sleeping in a chair next to my hospital bed. Barbara was working late, and she asked her to stay with me. My youngest daughter's day job was working for a real estate company whose president was auditioning to become the real estate version of *The Devil Wears Prada.*[4] As a result, her job was far more tiring than it should have been. And even though she lived in the city and her job was in downtown Chicago, she drove up to be with me. That night, as she sacked out in the chair, I slipped into and out of a light sleep. It was comforting to have her and her long brown hair curled up on the chair. We didn't need to talk. Her presence alone told me everything I needed to know.

As we were well into December, the rest of the world started getting excited about the holiday season with bits of Christmas and Hanukkah trappings popping up around our ward. Since the hospital stay put a crimp in my holiday shopping, I started to wonder if I could do all of my shopping online.

Other patients came and left. I memorized the food menu and got to know almost all my nurses on a first-name basis. I knew that my unflappable Bosnian nurse had arthritis in her right hand. I knew that the short Jamaican lady who made up my bed always had a 500 watt smile on her face. I knew that my marathoner nurse had graduated from University of Michigan and, before becoming a nurse, was a journalist in Israel. And I knew who was professionally cordial, who was genuinely interested in their patients and who stopped by to talk because they were a serial talker.

At night I pretended to sleep as I hoped that my newly scalped head and super-dooper antibiotics, would heal up, and waited.

Then one morning the Head of Neurosurgery popped into my room. After a perfunctory look at my head, he gave it to me straight, "We believe that your skull is infected. The only solution is to cut out the infected bone to protect the rest of your brain."

As I started to digest this news he then asked me "Have you had anything to eat this morning?" As it turns out, I love breakfast. As a kid growing up I watched a lot of Saturday morning kids' shows and those good folks at Kellogg have always told me how important it was to eat a good breakfast. I also believed that the breakfast put out by the kitchen at the hospital was their best meal of the day. Earlier that morning I scarfed down a scrumptious Denver omelet, crisp whole wheat toast, a tasty patty or two of breakfast sausage, a healthier fruit cup and washed it all down with several stiff cups of black coffee.

I relayed this to him and he was not particularly happy. He had wanted to operate on me that morning and wasn't available later in the day (it was against the rules to operate on someone with a full stomach).

He stomped about ten feet into the hallway where I heard him call one of his other staff surgeons from his cell phone and say something like "I wanted to operate on this guy, but he ate breakfast like a lumberjack! I'm out tomorrow. Can you operate on him tomorrow morning?"

As a result, I was then handed off to my third surgeon for my third trip to the operating room.

If memory serves me right, the odds are 50-50, in preparation for the surgery I needed to have some pre-operation tests. By now I was pretty familiar with the procedure: an orderly would wander up to your room with a gurney, you'd climb in and he'd wheel you off to some odd room in the sub-basement of the hospital.

For my craniectomy (the medical term for having part of your skull removed), I remember being woken up at 4 a.m. for a pre-surgery MRI. Few things are as quiet as a hospital at 4 a.m. Patients are sleeping. The halls are empty and dimly lit. The night shift nurses are huddled around computer screens doing paper work or, more likely, catching up on Facebook. Since this did anything but calm my nerves, I decided to take my mind off the impending operation by having some fun as I was being pushed around in the gurney.

I remembered what my buddy Greg told me about Indiana University football games, that every time the football team got a first down the entire stadium chanted the Dudley-Do-Right song for several bars as they made a locomotion-like motion with their arms. (Given the Indiana football team's sorry record of late, a first down is worth cheering.) So, of course, I decided to emulate the crowd. Every time we came up on a nurses' station, I'd start to move my arms in a locomotive like motion and sing the song: "Da, tada, ta, da, ta, da..."

The nurses would look up from their computer screens and stare at me. And listen. And stare some more. I'm sure some of them muttered, "I heard about that guy...brain tumor."

On the day of my "rear bone plate" skull removal surgery, i.e. the back of my skull that appeared infected, I was wheeled down to surgery on a gurney and parked in the "bullpen" area waiting for my third doctor (who was surprisingly conversational and unsurprisingly competent) to show up.

The bullpen is an area just outside the operating rooms where patients are stowed just before surgery. The rooms are separated by off-white curtains and often have small TVs in them for really long waits. My room provided partial views of several operating theaters. As you can imagine, it was as antiseptic visually as it was antiseptic medically. The walls looked sterile and either white or metallic.

The bullpen was rather cold which, I guessed, was to minimize the possibility of infection. A nice nurse came over, gave me a warm blanket and tucked the blanket snuggly around me. If I wasn't waiting to get my head sawed open, I would've enjoyed the sensation of being warm in the cold, much like the sensation of lounging in a hot tub after a day of skiing.

The medical staff wore white hairnets, off-green hospital gowns and tight facemasks that made them look a bit like bandits. There was little chatter and even fewer smiles. This was serious business being performed by serious professionals.

My new doctor was hung up with, I later learned, a bunch of paperwork. As I cooled my jets in the bullpen for what seemed like ages, I started to mentally walk through the events of the past week or so: waking up with an oozing head, seeing the infectious disease doctor, learning that *The Good Doctor* wouldn't be available to take care of me, being scalped and, now, preparing to have the infected portion of my skull sawed off.

Just as I was starting to feel sorry for myself, a young couple came down with their little girl. She was maybe four, maybe five years old with curly reddish shoulder-length hair. She was crying. She didn't like her hospital gown and kept trying to take it off. The operating arena with its bright lights and stark environment seemed to spook her.

I understood why this small, frightened girl was crying and squirming and holding onto her mother for dear life. The operating theater spooked me too. It reminded me of getting my tonsils out as a little kid and spending the night in the hospital. It was probably the first time I'd spent the night away from my parents or any close relative, and I didn't like it one bit.

Her parents were dressed in the same standard hospital-issued gowns and were trying to settle her down, but she wasn't having any of it. They cooed, they coddled and they hugged. Finally, she relaxed a wee bit and somebody slipped a gas mask on her. After a few breadths, she seemed to wilt and her parents walked out leaving her with the nurses.

I thought about her, her parents and the stress they were having. While I had no idea what kind of problem she had, my heart went out to all of them.

It was also a rather blatant lesson for me: if that couple and little girl with curly hair can go through this, I should veer off the self-pity path. One thing the hospital has nailed: the moment you start feeling sorry for yourself, you see another patient who has it far, far worse.

I reminded myself that I've had a very good life: great parents, a loving wife, terrific children. Tons of people would have loved to have lived my life. If this is the end, so be it. I said a prayer, doctor number three showed up, and I was wheeled into the operating room.

And while I looked, I didn't see a single radial arm saw.

When I woke up after the surgery, I found myself back in my room and saw that I had a massive gauzy white bandage wrapped around the top of my fragile head to protect my brain from, well, everything. My first thought was "It looks like I broke my head."

Back in grade school, when you had a broken arm or leg, everybody signed your cast and you got a lot of attention. In fact, if you didn't have a broken arm, you felt kinda jealous of all the attention the kid with the broken arm had. Everybody "Ooohed" and "Aaahed" and signed their cast. And while I didn't have a cast, I thought I could replicate the fun of having everybody sign something and I could still get a lot of attention.

So I asked my extremely competent, no-nonsense Bosnian nurse if I could have a roll of white tape for mental health purposes. After an overly long explanation on my part, and a meaningful stare on her part, she got me some from the supply room.

I then called Barbara and asked her to bring a magic marker to the hospital when she came to visit me.

With tape and magic marker in hand, I then asked every person who walked into my room to do two things: write their name and hometown down on a piece of tape, and *gently* stick it to my gauzy turban.

Everybody did. Folks wrote down places which included hometowns in Bosnia, Jamaica and Romania. Nurses who weren't assigned to me, but helped me during my previous operation, heard about my turban signing and made an effort to cruise into my room and sign it. The attention was wonderfully distracting as I tried hard not to thinking about my missing rear bone plate. In many ways it was "denial" at its best because I was too busy to have to invent stupid jokes.

Later in the day, a nurse from the infectious disease group barged into my room to check me out. She took a good long look at me and my gauze with all the tape and names. Her lips tightened into a short, thin grimace. Her forehead scrunched. Her nostrils flared and her face reddened. And then with her arms held straight in front of her and fingers extended, she read me the riot act: "What if the ink bleeds through the tape and gauze into your wound? This could very well compromise your wound when you are least able to protect yourself. I cannot believe the nurses in this ward allowed you to do this."

She was upset. She was aghast. She was indignant and self-righteous. I could've sworn that I was being lectured by somebody from the Women's Christian Temperance Union who just found a bunch of boys swigging beer in the church's basement. (And since the WCTU was founded not far from the hospital, she could very well have been a legacy member).

And while she didn't say so, I could just see her thinking: "I'm telling! I'm going to tell your infectious disease doctor and you are going to be in big trouble!" She reminded me of a particularly self-righteous tattle-tale from junior high who couldn't wait to "tell" when we switched seats on a substitute teacher in the 7th grade. And while I really wanted to stick my tongue out at her and reply in kind, I didn't.

Uncharacteristically, I took a deep breath, calmed myself and didn't utter a peep. It was hard, very hard and I think, a sign of increasing maturity, or some really potent drugs, that I didn't tell her that, if she looked closer, she would have seen my infectious disease doctor's signature on the lower right-hand side.

The Man in the Dorky Blue Mask

When I first woke up from surgery, one of the first questions the nurses asked me was "How are you going to make sure that you don't sleep on your brain?" It was also a tricky question.

Since my excised skull (i.e. cut-out bone) was in the lower left-hand section of the back of my skull, and I always sleep on my back, figuring out a safe way to sleep was a bit of a "sticky wicket." After a few delicate maneuvers, we decided that maybe I could sleep on my right side if we wedged several pillows behind my back to keep me from rolling onto my back in my sleep and squishing my unprotected brain.

Have you ever tried to change *how* you sleep? If you are a "side-sleeper" have you ever tried to sleep flat on your back? For me it's hard. I've always been a flat-back sleeper. Doesn't that lead to snoring you may ask? Not if you have a wife that jabs you with her (lovely and delicate) elbow as adroitly as Barbara does. I quickly learned to stop snoring or I'd be one of the "husband-abuse" cases you read about.

I also found out that my body started to give me all sorts of warning messages now that I didn't have a skull. A short walk down the hall gave me a dose of what to expect as my internal warning system told me to:

"Watch out for that 'Exit' sign" (five feet above my head)
"Be careful of the oxygen tank spigot behind you, you'd hate to bang your brains on that"!
"Whoa, what if that nurse down the hall turns around without looking and knocks you over?"

I certainly wasn't in any danger, but my body was nervous and worried. I kept getting these little reminders for months.

The day after surgery, my safety helmet was delivered. It was a dark navy blue, made of a sturdy yet pliable plastic material and about one half of an inch thick. It also had "air-holes" every few inches or so. This was the hospital-approved protective head gear for patients with a severe head injury or a piece of skull missing. It was also warmer than the warmest hat I'd ever worn. It was warmer than fur or down or some improbable combination of the two. I felt like I was in a sweatbox, after three minutes I was ready to spill my guts (I'd make a terrible spy):

"Do you want my social security number?"
"Can I give you the name of my contacts at HQ?"
"I'll tell you the secret handshake."
"Just please, please let me take this damned helmet off my head."

Nothing worked. The nurses told me to wear it when I went to sleep.

Now as a reminder, the ward was already pretty toasty. When you added this surgical helmet/mask, I was so hot I was sweating.

I would wake up in the middle of the night with the inside of the helmet caked with sweat. I'd take it off, wipe it off, put it back on and try to get another forty-five minutes or so of sleep before waking up again.

I quickly felt "at one" with *The Man in the Iron Mask.*[5]

I also wondered about how I'd fit into normal society. How could I attend a business conference or meeting? I tried to think of ways to make this funny and hide in denial:

"This is my homage to B.D. from the Doonesbury cartoon—he didn't take off his helmet either."
"This is actually the latest bike helmet style for the Tour de France."
"This is even warmer than those goofy-looking fur hats with the ear flaps."

I didn't laugh. No one else did either.

So we did the only thing possible. Barbara bought me a Chicago Bear's Santa hat to pull *over* the helmet. The combination focused everybody's eyes on Christmas and "'da Bears" instead of my dorky blue helmet. Conversations with nurses and visitors quickly tilted towards the Bears' prospects in the playoffs and Christmas lists.

Yes, I was hotter, but it was worth it.

During my second trip to the Evanston NorthShore Hospital, one of the "unspoken rules" of the hospital that bothered me was "don't talk to the orderlies while they're taking you someplace." I was taken from my room by orderlies to MRIs, X-rays, ultra-sounds and surgeries. Yet, I don't ever remember ever being introduced to one, "John, meet Mike, he's going to take you down to the operating theater." (That doesn't mean I wasn't introduced, it just means I don't *remember* being introduced.)

Even though I was often just partially awake, partially-drugged or fully drugged, it felt wrong to not at least introduce myself, so I'd say "Mike, I'm John, pleased to meet ya'. I'm wearing this goofy helmet so you can remember me among all the other patients you meet."

That wasn't exactly a sure-fire conversation starter, so through trial and error I learned that I could kick-off a conversation with just about anybody in the hospital by asking two questions:

"Where are you from?"
"What music do you like?"

I found out that the folks who worked at the Evanston Hospital made up one of the most international groups I had ever met. I talked to nurses, medical technicians and orderlies from Ireland, Kentucky, Turkey and a bunch of other foreign places I've forgotten.

My tried and true follow-up question to "where are you from" would be "what restaurant in Chicagoland serves the best Jamaican (or whatever country they were from) food and where is it?" I would then ask, "Why did you come here?" and "Why in the world did you come here from a warm climate, it's 7 degrees outside today and the wind chill is 20 below?"

My music question was especially fun as I got recommendations for gospel, jazz and reggae. My nurse with the 500-watt smile would get this little glow in her eyes when she started to talk about "real" gospel music. One of my nurses was married to a bandleader. Before I left she brought me a CD of her husband's band, *I Will Never Stop Loving You* by Charley Organaire & Sunshine Festival, and I gave her a Chicago Bear's Santa hat.

Yes, I got the better gift.

I went back and read a note I sent to myself on Wednesday, December 12th. It started out saying "Yesterday was the worst day of the second (hospital) stay." The email then reminded me that, on Tuesday, they started the day by taking out my shunt which I always thought of as my "drainage pipe."

Now think back to that time when you visited the "Our Body" exhibit at your local museum which showed the two lobes of the brain. If you can't remember, go online and look at some picture. *The Good Doctor*, or perhaps one of her minions, stuck this shunt in-between the two halves of my brain so the edema (swelling caused by excess fluid trapped in my body's tissue) could drain before it squashed my brain, or even splashed my brain. Before I went home, however, they needed to remove the "shunt" and close the wound.

That morning a confident, young and well-coiffed doctor waltzed into my room and told me that she needed to perform this minor procedure. I pulled off my miserably hot dorky blue helmet so she could initiate this little procedure. When she started to pull out the shunt, I felt like it was located at the very core of my "being." I could never remember feeling anything so deep inside my head. It was unnerving.

She then needed to close the wound. I think I said, "So, you're going to give me a couple of stitches, huh?" I was used to stitches. I had stitches all over my head. I knew what to expect from stitches.

Yes, it's time for another pop quiz. Pick one:

A. She effectively gave me a face lift by pulling so hard on my stitches.
B. She used "super glue" instead of stitches to bind my wound.
C. She used Elmer's Glue which is almost as good and a lot cheaper.
D. She stapled my head.

Yes, she picked "D." She stapled my head. She may have said something like, "the doctor prefers staples." I thought, "Staples? Surely you've got to be joking." She wasn't joking; she wasn't Shirley; and she quickly shot a staple into my head, BAM.

That hurt. That hurt more than any other medical procedure for which I was awake. Now based on my standing in the "Professional Patients of America," this broke one of the most sacred rules in the patient-medical profession code of engagement; early warning of in-coming pain. I thought all medical professionals, no matter how well-coiffed, were honor-bound to *warn* you when something was going to hurt. That way you could ask for a shot of whiskey, gird-your-loins or do some pre-emptive sniveling.

I tried to look at her but she deftly hid behind me. And then without any warning, "BAM," she stapled me again. I thought Guy Fieri was somewhere in the room doing color commentary and snickering.ᵉ

She covered her face and ran out of the room as best she could in her high heels. I don't remember an "I'm sorry" or "you'll feel better quickly" or even a "better you than me."

I was feeling the pain. I was mad. I was sick and tired of being a good soldier. I was sick and tired of being sick and tired. I was out of jokes and out of patience. I felt like my body had been cut, shot, and hacked apart...and indeed it had. I was on the edge of just losing it, of falling into some deep black enormous psychic bottomless well of self-pity that, once in, would be awfully hard to climb out of. I felt like an over-burdened camel on spindly legs trying to dodge that last bit of straw. As I was soon to find out, that last bit of straw landed on me later that afternoon.

Following the resection of my infected skull, my infectious disease doctor ran a bunch of tests to determine the best antibiotic for my pesky infection. For my infection I learned that I would need to be on antibiotics for six weeks. Sounds simple, right? To cure this particular infection, however, the antibiotics dosage took an hour to administer, and needed to be administered every four hours around the clock. Who can change IV bags every four hours for weeks at a time? You'd be exhausted and never be able to do this at home.

The ingenious medical solution is a PIC line, a "personal intravenous catheter" line. It's a teeny, tiny thin tube that is inserted into your vein and travels about forty-five centimeters (roughly 17 inches or so) into your body towards your heart. The other end sticks out of your vein (somewhere a bit north of your elbow) and has a nozzle on it that allows the caretaker to easily attach and detach an IV. The IV is attached to a small, pre-programmed machine that automatically injects the antibiotics into your body.

The key to making this all work is inserting the PIC line into the patient in the first place. I was assured that inserting the PIC line was safe, easy to insert and relatively painless. In fact, I wouldn't even need to have any anesthetic. Having just had my head stapled, though, my BS antenna was tuned to "high" and this fluid explanation just sounded a little too simple. According to the nurse who came to brief me, the procedure would be done in my own hospital bedroom and it would take longer to set-up than actually perform the procedure.

Let's review the scorecard, up until now I:

Had a craniotomy to remove the tumor (or at least part of the tumor),
Been scalped,
Had a craniectomy to remove the infected piece of my skull,
Fell into the *Bottom 10%*,
Had up to three IVs stuck in me at once,
Was stapled without warning, and…
…was on day ten of what was supposed to be a three day hospital stay during the Christmas season.

None of these upset me like the thought of a tube going up my vein. I don't know if it was the "straw that broke the camel's back" or just the idea of having a tube in my vein. I didn't like it. I wasn't gonna like it. And I couldn't wait to get done with it.

Having had the shitty shunt experience, I could only imagine what this was really going to be like. While waiting for the team to show up, I tried to steady my nerves by keeping busy. I tried to get my Lumosity scores up into double digits. I wiped my sweaty brow. I wrestled a "one star" Sudoku puzzle (and gave up). I ordered a stir-fry lunch, which seemed like the healthiest thing on the menu, and pushed everything around my plate two or three times. And I tried to meditate, except I didn't really know how to meditate.

I had started watching HGTV and just began to fantasize about buying a waterfront condo in Belize when two very competent-looking, veteran medical nurses arrived and proceeded to prep the room. They shut the door and, I think, put up a "Do Not Disturb" sign.

At first they were all business. They put down fresh linen, raised the bed to about five feet off the ground (through some fancy hydraulic system in the bed) and started to prep my arm. They also set up some special equipment (gamma-ray goggles? A portable X-ray machine? Who knew?) that would let them track their progress.

I tried to lie very still in my dorky blue helmet as they began to insert the tubing into my vein with the aid of some contraption I couldn't quite see. As they did it, I couldn't avoid hearing a conversation between the two of them that went something like this:

> "This is the longest PIC line I think I've ever seen!"
> "I'll bet you I could jump rope with this thing."
> "You aren't going to…"
> ""Just watch! Raspberry, strawberry, apple jam tart. Tell me the name of your sweet heart."
> "Now stop that, I go on break in 5 minutes."
> "Girls just want to have fun…" (sung)
> "I'll drive and you guide."
> "Halfway, now are we going to take the left fork or the right fork?"
> "Beats me, did you bring a map?"

"Map? Are you living in the dark ages? I use a GPS, honey."

"Here, let me flip a coin—heads is the right fork and tails is left."

"It's tails, take the left fork."

"Well, would you look at that, the entire vein just collapsed?!"

"Should we pull out and start over again?"

"Yeah, I guess we have to back up a ways."

"Do these veins look congested or is it just me?"

"I'll put in a ticket for Roto-Rooter after we're done."

"Okay, let's try the right vein."

"Now, I think we're finished."

"Let me take a look with the supersonic X-ray vision goggles."

"I've seen worse, we're done."

I was awake the entire time and never felt like such an inconsequential bystander when somebody was working on my body. I didn't have the "rear bone plate" of my skull, I still had a sizeable chunk of tumor and now I also had a tube running up my vein. That's it, I wanted out. I'm pretty sure they wanted me out, too.

Outside the weather was cold, windy and slick. Inside, I was similarly frosted. I sat there in my room wearing my dorky blue helmet and sulked. I sulked about having my skull cut out. I sulked about landing in the *Bottom 10%*. I sulked about being in the hospital for the tenth day in a row. I sulked about having a PIC line stuck up my vein.

I sat in my bed, wore my dorky blue helmet and asked the nurses to shut my door and, essentially, put that "Do Not Disturb" sign back up.

Pretty soon the lady who took our meal orders came into my room and shut the door. She was short and well-groomed with a stylish corn-row hair style. She always seemed attentive without being overly nosy or pushy.

I was not interested in ordering dinner. I was not interested in chatting. I wanted to be alone, and sulk and wallow in my misery.

She then softly, gently and quietly told me that she, too, had a brain tumor. Unlike me, though, she'd had multiple complex operations. I forget how many operations she had, but it seemed like at least four, and maybe more like six.

She pointed to her head and bowed down so I could see her scars.

Looking as closely as I dared, well, she won the scars contest. It seemed like she had a crazy-quilt of scars, a skull assembled from the remnants of several different leftover skulls that somehow, someway got patched into hers.

How did she know to come see me? Was she some sort of angel sent to remind me that my situation could be a lot worse? Was she sent here by the nurses to tell me to "suck it up?" "Was she just some caring, thoughtful person?"

The more I tried to grapple with these issues, the more I got wrapped around my own axel. The only cogent conclusion I came to was that I ought to be happy with what I've got. It's a hard lesson to learn, especially when you're wearing a dorky blue helmet.

I mumbled something vague and inappropriate, and she tenderly closed the door and left.

On Wednesday, the day I hoped to leave, *The Good Doctor* returned from her overseas trip and visited me as part of her usual rounds. I was sitting in bed, wearing my dorky blue helmet and wrestling a "Find the Word" puzzle rehab assignment when she walked in looking like a million bucks and a commanding general all rolled into one.

She looked at me and quizzically said "Why are you wearing that helmet in bed?"

I gasped. My eyes bulged a bit. My brows made furrows so deep you could plant corn.

I finally wheezed out something like "because everybody has told me that I have to wear this (dorky blue) helmet 24 hours a day until I get my skull fixed."

She might have then asked "are you having trouble walking?" I said "no," and told her that my balance was just fine, thank you; and I that probably logged upwards of a mile a day in the hallways of our ward.

In a nearly scolding tone she then said "You only need to wear that in the car in case you get into an accident."

The clouds parted, angels sang and the music swelled. At that moment I knew there really was a wonderful, munificent God who truly did "watch over his flock."

5

Home Alone

WINTER HAD KICKED INTO AN EVEN HIGHER GEAR by the time I got home on December 14th. Outside temperatures rarely got out of the twenties. It had snowed, and at that time, four to six inches of snow on the ground seemed like a lot. We have a one hundred and twenty year old house and it's drafty. I was convinced that a lit match would be blown out if you held it up to several leaky spots in the house. And with the winter solstice just around the corner, it seemed dark outside all the time.

It was dark on the inside too, as Louis had declined in health since I'd been at the hospital. Once the fastest and friskiest dog on the beach, he now slept a lot more than usual and struggled uncomfortably to get to his feet on our the slick hardwood floors. We started putting throw rugs all over the house just so he could get his footing. The vet put him on a pain killer and doggie glucosame for his joints, so I added him to the daily medication schedule. He'd also become "untrained" during my absence. Each night Barbara and I would worry about him having an accident (the odds seemed to be 50-50).

At some level I was thankful that I was home. On another level I was still spooked by my on-going skull infection. On a third level I was trying to show everybody that I was going to be all right. I'm not sure I believed that, but I was trying to put on a brave front.

We still expected ten guests or so to show up for dinner on Christmas day, and wanted to make sure that we could still roll out a reasonable feast along with everybody's favorite Christmas cookies. Usually we have a massive Christmas cookie decorating event in which everybody gets a little too competitive about who has the best decorated cookie. We usually kick-off the decorating by putting out several boxes of Christmas cookie forms, different frosting colors and variously colored sprinkles for decoration. Some years, we'd take pictures of our collective best efforts and I'm sure Barbara posted some winners on Facebook.

But, both Barbara and I were significantly behind our decorating, gift-buying and Christmas cheer in general. We decided to "skinny-down" our holiday commitments: Barbara would make fewer cookies, we'd eliminate the competitive cookie trimming, we'd hang fewer decorations and we'd get a smaller tree. Given my condition, I planned on ordering almost all my presents through gift catalogs.

And, while we were both trying to catch up with the holiday season, we also had to get used to our new best friend, my new mobile IV.

Soon after we got home from the hospital, my home nurse (who would be visiting me once a week) and a representative of the home care company came to our house to show Barbara and me how to operate the pre-programmed mini-computer and change the IV. Both the antibiotics and minicomputer would be inserted into a black nylon bag that looked suspiciously like a *French Male Purse*, only not as fashionable.

Actually, first they tried to teach themselves how to use the device and, in the process, totally confused and frightened both of us. As they experimented with the device we learned that neither of them had *actually* used this model and, of course, there weren't any handy directions written down for us to use.

I made a mental note to figure out who the bright product manager for this high-tech, totally un-user-friendly product was and send him some uncensored customer feedback. Had he been within arm's reach, I would have left my own personalized version of braille notes on his neck. (If he was a "her," I'd let Barbara do the strangling.)

That night, after the 10 p.m. news, I climbed upstairs, brushed my teeth and climbed into bed with my new best friend, my *French Male Purse*. Our sleeping arrangements became strategic. Since the surgery was primarily on the lower-left hand back side of my head, I needed to sleep on my right side and prop up my back with pillows so I didn't roll onto my back when I was asleep (which I longed to do) and squash my unprotected brain. I then placed the *French Male Purse* in front of my chest on the bed. As I never sleep on my stomach, that seemed like a safe place to put it.

I then tried to go to sleep which was still a bit of a challenge.

Since Barbara is a David Letterman fan and a night-owl, she probably climbed into bed a several hours later.

What happened next is a bit of a blur, but I think that, almost immediately after she climbed into bed, I started to get a dose. While I couldn't feel the antibiotics being pumped into my arm, I could hear the machine "whirring." The whirring was a rather mechanical and a new mechanical sound in our very quiet bedroom which I found hard to ignore. I listened to this new sound rather intently until it stopped. If memory serves me right, the mini-computer proudly "honked" once when it was done pumping. If you hadn't already been awake, it woke you up.

Gee, thanks, I needed that.

Maybe an hour or so later, an alarm went off: "BEEP, BEEP, BEEP." Both Barbara and I jerked ourselves awake. What was wrong? It wasn't my alarm clock. It wasn't Barb's alarm clock. It wasn't the fire alarm. We didn't have a burglar alarm...it was the *French Male Purse*.

Beep! Beep! Beep!

Damn, what's wrong? I tried to turn on the lamp on my nightstand and nearly knocked it over. Once on, I zipped open the *French Male Purse* case and tried to read the computer's alarm code on the machine. Since I didn't have my glasses on, I couldn't read anything.

Ok, where were my glasses? Weren't they on the nightstand?

Beep! Beep! Beep!

Barbara said "What's wrong?" I said "Something's wrong with the *French Male Purse* and I can't find my glasses." Louis heard the commotion and barked.

I crawled around on the floor looking for my glasses that I obviously knocked off the nightstand. Since I was focused on finding my glasses, I yanked the *French Male Purse* with my beeping mini-computer off the bed. It fell to the ground with a "thud."

Beep! Beep! Beep!

What if I broke it? These things must cost a fortune. How would I get dosed tonight? Would this screw up everything?

Barbara said "Do you need help?" What I really needed was to have a close and personal closed-door conversation with the *French Male Purse* product manager.

Beep! Beep! Beep!

I found my glasses, opened up the *French Male Purse* and read the error code on the mini-computer: "Kink in line." I straightened out the line. It stopped beeping. This time I put the bag on the nightstand so my tossing and turning wouldn't kink the line. We turned out the lights and tried to go to sleep.

Maybe two hours later the alarm sounded again: Beep! Beep! Beep!

This time I was better organized: I turned on the light without smacking the lamp or knocking my glasses halfway across the room. I opened the *French Male Purse* and tried to figure out what was wrong.

Beep! Beep! Beep!

I looked at the error code, checked the line and was baffled. I started randomly pushing buttons which did no good at all. So I did what any software guy would do, I rebooted the mini-computer, which then worked just fine.

It was maybe 3:30 or 4 a.m.. We both pretended to go to sleep for the next couple of hours. I finally gave up and waddled downstairs around 5 a.m. or so and fed Louis. We'd survived the first night.

The next night we changed the IV bag before I went to sleep. This was a little bit like changing a newborn baby. We reread our handwritten directions several times before starting. We disinfected our hands. And we handled the mini-computer and bag of antibiotics very, very carefully.

I felt that Barbara and I were reliving some strange reenactment of the movie *Kramer versus Kramer* when the father and son can't even make pancakes. Or maybe we were stuck in our own version of the movie, *Groundhog Day,* and were doomed to flounder in bed night after night until we figured out how to do this correctly.

Later, we had another kinked line and another mystery "Beep!" that I, again, rebooted.

On the third night the battery died. Apparently the mysterious "Beep! Beep! Beep!" was announcing a dying battery, or at least that's what I thought it was. This caused a variety of worries: would the revived micro-computer know where it was in the dosing cycle when the battery died? Would I be "overdosed?" I changed the batteries and everything worked just fine (I decided not to strangle the product manager just yet.)

This is how we learned to change the batteries on a daily basis. And guess what, the home care company had given us enough batteries to do so although I don't remember being instructed to do so.

I mentally hit myself on the forehead like Homer ("Duh"!).

Now that we had used "trial and error and error" to educate ourselves, we were the "Pro's from Dover."[2] Better than that, we were the father and son from *Kramer versus Kramer* at the *end* of the movie. We changed IV bags, slapped in new batteries and caught up on sleep. Well, Barbara caught up on sleep; I still woke up at strange hours of the morning from one of several meds messing with my mind.

Somewhere close to the two week mark, I got a phone call from my infectious disease doctor.

"John?"

"Yes?"

"This is your infectious disease doctor."

"Yes?" (I was still on heavy drugs and not a dapper conversationalist.)

"We just found out that you are also infected with some slow growing, non-oxygen bacteria."

"Yes?"

"So we need to change your antibiotic to one that will also kill this newly found problem."

"Yes?"

"So we are going to send you out a new antibiotic solution today."

"Yes?"

"The good news is that you won't have to be hooked up to the machine twenty-four hours a day."

"Yessss?"

"You will only need to hook up a syringe to your PIC line and be dosed twice a day."

"Yes?"

"You want to kill *all* the infection, right?"

"Yes."

"But you will have to start a new six week cycle of dosing to make sure you're cured."

"This is a joke, right?"

It wasn't a joke. Later that day the new antibiotics and syringes and assorted medical stuff were delivered. My home stay nurse came over and showed Barbara how to attach the syringe to the PIC line and "shoot me up."

About this time I started to worry about getting a job sometime, somehow, somewhere. Probably more accurately, I was worried about getting any job, at any company, at any time. Given that in January 2011 the country seemed to be in the worse economic times since the Great Depression, employers could afford to be very picky.

I tried to use the old sports trick of envisioning a successful job interview: seeing it, smelling it, feeling it. I imagined walking into the office of a successful company in the suburbs, waiting patiently in the artfully decorated lobby and then being shown into a stark, windowless interview room by a competent but not particularly talkative receptionist. I then saw myself meeting and shaking hands with a tough, dour-faced personnel director and having a conversation that went something like this:

"Well Mr. Kerastas what is this blank spot in your resume during the 4th Quarter?"

"I had a health issue."

"What kind of health issue?"

"I had a brain tumor."

"Are you cured?"

"Not totally, the surgery removed 70% of the tumor, but I still have to go through 'completion' surgery and radiation treatments."

"No problem, half the people around here are brain dead anyway."

"Our office is about 35 miles from your house and nowhere near public transportation, do you have a car?"

"I do have a car, but my occupational therapist hasn't cleared me for driving yet."

"No problem, we have a group which car pools from your area and I'm sure they'd like to have somebody else to split the cost with them."

"Do you have any industry experience?"

"Absolutely none."

"That's even better! You have no bad habits to unlearn."

"What is your most profitable product?"

"Our competition claims that our most profitable product contains a known carcinogen, can you turn a blind eye to that?"

"The tumor left me only 25% blind in my right eye, so I can't turn an *entirely* blind eye to it."

"Well Mr. Kerastas that would be a problem for us."
"But I'm a bit blind in my left eye, too!"
"Don't call use, we'll call you."

In writing this, I've asked myself, "Why, WHY am I concocting, telling or regurgitating all these bad jokes?" At the time I thought it was a defense mechanism, but actually, it was just another form of denial. By joking with friends, family and myself about *The Blob*, I could try to *deny* its seriousness and its repercussions.

Right around this time my mother sent me an article from *the Detroit News* that said, "Survival after diagnosis is improving: More than 31% of patients are alive five years later, up from 21% in the 1990s."[3]

That was a pretty sobering statistic: *only* 310 of 1,000 brain tumor victims are still alive after five years? A score of .310 is a good batting average if you're a professional baseball player but it isn't a life expectancy I was all that excited about. (I'm still hoping that those of us with meningioma do much, much better than the overall average.)

Growing up in the '50s, I often heard that real men, brave men "laugh in the face of danger." There is an aspect of that—the tall, dark, handsome, movie-star version—that I find totally disconnected from reality. From what I can tell from talking to WWII or Vietnam veterans, men who know what war or danger is all about are scared down to their toes. If you aren't scared, you don't really understand the situation. To my way of thinking, courage is doing the right thing even when you have the snot scared out of you.

Let me make this crystal clear: I have no snot. It's all been scared right out of me. Each bump in this seemingly endless pot-hole-ridden, brain-tumor littered road is unnerving. My weak attempts at humor are even weaker attempts at dodging the real issues that I feel are being thrown in my face: loss of competence, loss of spousal appeal, loss of any patriarchal role, loss of self-respect.

And here's the kicker: I have it good, real good. I have a loving wife, great kids, terrific friends, supportive church buddies and what passes for financial security in this day and age. I can only imagine what it's like to have a more aggressive brain tumor and to be fighting this disease without friends, family and church behind you. My imagination tells me that would be a living nightmare.

My suspicions were confirmed when I started reading what I can only describe as an entire tribe of brutally honest, utterly defiant and powerfully angry brain tumor and cancer bloggers. They were sick, they were mad and they were going to tell the world how they felt.

My first experience with the online brain tumor community was with the *It's Just Benign* which is a website exclusively dedicated to victims and relatives or friends of meningioma victims. The site lets everybody post all sorts of questions for help or information or, sometimes, just a sympathetic ear. I'd read postings where folks asked for advice on surgical techniques, or prayers for young children with recurrent tumors or treatment for victims that survived surgery but were left with paralyzed legs. Somehow my problems, even with my infected skull, seemed small compared to their desperate situations.

I then started reading different brain tumor and cancer blogs. The blogs I admired the most had a savage, take-no-prisoners edge to them, like Kalin Marie's blog, *Cancer is Hilarious* (which, of course, means it's not). She wrote with intimacy and rage and honesty that made me feel like she was talking to her best friend over a cup of coffee.

In another corner of the same emotional sandbox, Amy Marash wrote and drew a blog entitled *Cancer Is So funny*. She poured emotions into sketches that defined her black feelings in ways that words just can't quite capture.

I then stumbled across *Fuck Cancer and the horse it rode in on*. The blog's URL tells you something too: http://baldylocks.blogspot.com. The "Stupid Cancer Rant" video she posted captured her bubbling emotional cocktail of rage, anguish and bravado in a way that just cracked me up. It adroitly walks the fine line between comedy and tragedy.

One line that has stuck with me, though, is from *All Lie of the Mind* in which blogster Samantha Kittle writes, "Brain tumors are funny, but they're not hilarious." I remember it because it is not only bitingly sardonic, but it also leverages another meaning of "funny" which, according to the Merriam-Webster dictionary, is "differing from the ordinary in a suspicious, perplexing, quaint or eccentric way." That resonated with me. I have found my brain tumor to be both suspicious and perplexing.

These blogs showed that some victims knew how to experience the pain, accept their handicaps and start to emotionally invest themselves in their "new normal" and "move on." I hadn't figured that out yet.

At the same time I started reading these blogs, I was also on my new antibiotic regimen. This regimen consisted of two doses a day, twelve hours apart. Since I couldn't screw the antibiotic injection to my PIC line by myself, Barbara had to apply the dose, i.e. shoot me up (Have I mentioned how versatile she is?)

We settled on a 7 a.m. and 7 p.m. schedule for the antibiotics. That way Barbara could shoot me up before work, and again after coming home from work without having to "stick" me.

Now you may say, "Huh? What do you mean "stick?" Well, for those of you who haven't been sick lately, "stick" is the new term for "shot." For example, a nurse might say, "we are going to give you a little stick right here in your thigh for your morning Keppra dose." Or some medical professional might say, "We're going to give you a little stick of some topical anesthetic before the basil cell procedure, it won't hurt at all."

You may further ask yourself, "is that really true?" The answer is:

A. Of course it's true, a licensed and fully-trained medical professional just told you.
B. Well, it's partially true, think twice about the "not hurting" bit.
C. Lies! Lies! Lies!
D. Yes, it's true. They will give you a shot.

The answer is "D." Whether or not it hurts is irrelevant to the fact that you are about to get a needle thrust right into your body: sometimes your arm, occasionally your shoulder and, every once and a while, in your stomach (which always freaked me out). If the nurse is competent, had a full night's sleep, and isn't mad at the last patient, it may not hurt too badly.

The best part of having a PIC line is that you are not "stuck" every time you need an injection. Unless the injector is in a hurry and stomps on the syringe, you hardly feel it at all. In fact, it's more like having a vial of antibiotics hooked up to your very own personal garden hose. The hose, then, is used to squirt the antibiotics into your vein. Hmmm, that analogy doesn't seem to work at all.

Maybe a better analogy is getting fuel at the gas station. In this case, you are the car, and the antibiotics are stored in the gas pump. Personally, I kept asking for the highest octane (91), but I think Barbara put me down for 87 octane which was a lot cheaper.

Even though the PIC line was easy to use, the every twelve hour timing became a problem. I am an "early bird" and have been known to go to 6 a.m. group workouts at the gym.

Barbara, on the other hand, is a night owl; and at 9 p.m. she's at the peak of her game just as I start to yawn. Perhaps a better description is that Barbara's body clock is set for the Pacific Time Zone; mine is set for the Eastern Time Zone; and we both live together in the Central Time Zone.

So what? The "what" is that the 7 p.m. antibiotic dosing was no problem, we were both wide awake. The early morning infusion, however, was a bit of a trial.

There is a certain pathetic-ness to gently nudging your wife in the morning and saying "Sorry for waking you, Hon', it's time for my meds... would you shoot me up?" She's not happy about being woken up so early, is genuinely struggling to wake up, but knows she needs to do so. I felt like a junkie.

I said to myself, "How would a real "man" address his wife in the morning?" "Rise and shine! Get your butt in gear! Hurry! Hurry! Hurry! What are going to do? Lie around all day? Time to jump out of bed, put on your nurse's outfit and shoot me up."

I could then imagine her delicately but forcefully explaining that me and my antibiotics could "take a long walk off a short pier."

The 7 p.m. infusion also became somewhat of a road block to any sort of social life like 7 p.m. movie showings, 7 p.m. dinners with friends and early evening dinner parties ("Please excuse me and my wife while she gives me my meds, you can watch if you want.").

We did this for six sleepy-eyed weeks.

In late January, we had a bit of a thaw; and then temperatures quickly dropped turning the entire north shore into an icy *Slip 'n Slide* which made walking especially dicey. So I stayed inside and felt trapped.

While that seemed bad at the time, the weather got worse—much worse. On January 31st, over 20 inches of snow fell by midday. Our children had varying degrees of difficulty getting back to their own apartments. Our youngest daughter was stuck in a bus on Lake Shore Drive, but didn't get caught in the highly publicized traffic jam that snared hundreds of cars and, I guess, thousands of people. The vicious wind made our old house wheeze and crack, and our furnace battled to keep us warm. In the living room it was pretty toasty and I could feel like the furnace won. If I sat in the family room which had glass windows on three sides, I felt like winter weather had won as we'd dive under some blankets or pile on several ancestral Afghans to keep from freezing as we watched TV.

Louis' health took another step downhill. His back legs seemed even weaker and more arthritic. He continued to have "accidents" in the house. His energy level waned. There was nothing about this that cheered me up. It made me wonder if I was on the same downhill slide—a slide that would take me from energetic middle-aged man to a low-energy old codger.

This wondering helped motivate me to renew my rehab efforts and climb out of the *Bottom 10th percentile*.

Repeating my previous anal behavior, I developed a spreadsheet to track my efforts. I wanted to spend at least six hours a day working on rehab. During those six hours I wanted to tackle at least 10 Lumosity brain exercises, do all the visual exercises that my occupational therapist had given me, complete a *Circle-the-Word* game, complete a *Can you spot the differences? Life Magazine* puzzle and, with luck, finish one other exercise. I created a spreadsheet to keep track of my daily Keppra dosages, Louis' meds and my rehab activities in an effort to document my rehab work and make sure I was taking my meds.

After one rehab session, my therapist gave me some new harder *Circle-the-Word* exercises. So the next day after a hot breakfast on another cold winter day, I took a cup of steaming hot coffee with me into the living room where I plunked myself down into our comfy, faux-leather chair to tackle this new assignment. In "Circle-the-word" exercises, which you can buy in most book stores, I'd look at a sheet of letters laid on a grid that were fifteen letters across and fifteen letters down, seemingly listed in an arbitrary fashion. Each puzzle, however, would have fifteen to thirty or so words "hidden" within them. The words might read top to bottom, bottom to top, side to side, inverted or reverted (whatever that means). For this new harder assignment, each individual page took me over five hours (she asked me to keep track of the amount time spent on all three of them). It was a brutal reminder that I hadn't recovered from the operation, that I was in the *Bottom 10%*, and that I wasn't yet "normal."

A frustrating reality of rehab was that nobody could tell me what I could achieve if I gave maximum effort. Apparently a brain injury can't be reduced to an equation like "100 hours of rehab equals a 15 to 20% improvement." It might be that "100 hours of rehab equals no improvement at all."

At some level, actually at many levels, this annoyed me. If rehab was so important, why can't I have some clue as to my potential cognitive recovery? If I couldn't be my original 100%, could I get to 90%? 75%? Do I hear a bid for 60%?

On the other hand, it initially seemed pretty clear that no effort would result in no improvement, or would it? Part of me wondered that if I just gave my brain time to heal, how close to my previous intelligence level could I get?

While it might just work, I had too much of a puritan upbringing to just sit around and do nothing. So I continued to wrestle the exercises. While I would have good days and bad days, over the weeks I slowly climbed out of the *Bottom 10%* to the 20s, the 30s and beyond.

Sometime in January, we had a check-up appointment with *The Good Doctor*. While snow still covered the ground, we'd gotten used to it. The streets were clear and the snow made everything look clean and tidy. At the appointment she reiterated that she was going to wait another couple of months or so before "completion surgery."

There were two steps to completion surgery. The first step would be replacing the missing bone in my head so that I had an entire, water-proof and bump-resistant skull. That could either be by reinserting my old rear bone plate piece (post-deep freeze to kill the non-oxygen germs) or replacing it with an artificial prosthetic skull. I wasn't quite sure how she was going to decide which option was best and didn't really care. While it was my head, it was her expertise; and why would I argue with her? I knew nothing about patching skulls.

I was more worried about the second procedure, radiation. At that time, she was leaning towards giving me five treatments on an every-other-day basis. For some reason, the idea of radiation made me a lot more nervous than reinserting my old, disinfected skull. I could relate to cleaning off something, like a piece of wood in the deck, and nailing it back into place. If it didn't fit, you could take it out, sand down the offending side a bit, and slide it back into place. Radiation didn't seem to have that "do over" option. Once you were blasted, you glowed.

I had a cousin who had radiation treatments. Afterwards, she wasn't supposed to get near her husband for some time for fear of radiating him. I thought if it was that bad for him, how bad was it for her? Barbara had a sister who swallowed a radiation pill that was designed to kill her dysfunctional thyroid. After taking it, her husband was banned from being in the same room with him until she passed the pill. Wait, that doesn't sound right. Maybe she had to wait until she stopped glowing and couldn't read in bed without a night light? Whatever the reason and time period, neither of these sounded like something I wanted to go or glow through.

As she usually did, though *The Good Doctor* made both procedures sound like they were rather common, low risk events.

She also murmured rather positively about my wound, its appearance and our strategy of letting the tumor shrink some more before radiation treatments.

Then she asked if we had any questions. I said I was tackling rehab with a vengeance, and, other than not being able to sleep on my back and the resulting problems sleeping, had no complaints.

She stood up and her five foot or so frame seemed to grow to six foot four inches. She had an odd yet determined look on her face and said "you can sleep on your back." (I don't remember the rest of her comments other than maybe something about staying away from archery ranges.)

Once again I could've sworn I heard a choir of angels, felt a white spotlight shine down from the heavens and started to have this goofy smile on my face. I'm sure *The Good Doctor* thought this a rather strange reaction, but didn't pry.

I looked at Barbara. She looked, knowingly, at me. I wasn't sleepy at all, but I couldn't wait to go home and go to bed.

That first night was a bit eerie. For the first time in weeks, if not months, I laid down on my back and the only thing protecting my brain from the pillow was my skin and a few strands of hair. Nothing hurt, but I got the uncomfortable sensation that I was compressing my brains. It seemed like I could sort of feel the edges of partially numb bone around the wound pushing into the pillow. In the middle of that wound was an eerily empty area in which felt almost nothing. Ugh. So I lay on my back but turned my head somewhat to the right, which mitigated the "brain-compression" feeling. I continued this uneasy dance with my pillow until after "completion" surgery was completed.

Sometime in February, I finished my antibiotic regimen. Freed from the tyranny of every twelve hour injections, we started to go out more. We went to basketball games, concerts and the like. I learned how to scan through my blind spots and walk in crowds without knocking over little old ladies or my wife (her elbows were still pretty sharp). Everyday Louis and I would go for a walk, sometimes two or three walks. Part of this walking was a craving for exercise. Another part of it was trying to avoid an old dog having an accident. And part of it was an attempt to show myself, and the world, that I was bound and determined to maximize my new normal.

No matter how cold or snowy it was outside, Louis loved to get out and walk. Even though there was nothing to smell and little to see under the foot or so of snow lying around, he loved to walk. And I loved to walk with him (even if our pace slowed down to a crawl given his gimpy legs).

During those cold, windy walks, the helmet was pretty helpful. While it was crazy hot to wear in the hospital, it was comfortably warm outdoors in ten degree weather over a knit hat. I wore it everywhere I went: on walks, on car rides and on the train.

There was something wonderfully secure about wearing that helmet. It made me believe that, even if I did fall on some hidden piece of ice, I'd be alright. If we got into a car accident, I'd probably be just fine. Linus had his security blanket and I had my blue foam helmet.

That's when I became concerned that I had developed an unnatural attachment to the helmet. I became overly protective of it. People would say "Why don't you put a decal on it?" I'd stiffen and felt like saying, half-jokingly, "the HELMET's offended by the idea of such a desecration."

I have a fuzzy memory of Barbara gently asking me if I really needed to wear it while walking to a local restaurant from our car when the sidewalks were bone dry and clear of any snow or ice. I paused, thought about it, and started to worry if I was becoming psychologically warped like the guys in those movies where the ventriloquist's dummy would start giving orders to the ventriloquist. So I gently left the helmet in the car and walked to the restaurant without wearing it and my helmet didn't even complain...much.

One of the best rehab assignments that my favorite therapist gave me was to plan a trip from my home in the Chicago area to the west coast. I guess she wanted to see if I could figure out how to use Google maps and make a realistic plan, one that didn't have me driving fifteen hundred miles a day to get to the beach in Santa Clara.

So the next morning I sat at my desk in the attic to sort out this assignment. We'd rehabbed the third-floor attic years ago and it was a pleasantly secluded spot where you could see over most of the houses in the neighborhood. Unlike most of the rest of the house, it had plush carpeting and steeply pitched roofs of which I had become keenly aware, for potential head banging possibilities, as I walked towards my desk. It was also quiet. Since Louis wasn't allowed above the first floor, I was all alone in the attic.

The biggest downside to the attic was no heat, none. So even with the door to the attic open to let in every possible bit of warm air, it often seemed to be hovering close to sixty degrees which isn't bad if you're playing football, but rather frosty if you're sitting down and doing Lumosity. On the coldest days I just gave up and worked at the kitchen table. For Christmas, Barb had given me wool gloves with the tips of the fingers cut off as kind of a joke, but I used them and needed them.

As I sat in the attic, I first thought that this was one of those deadly dull assignments where I'd have to plan routes to cities I've never been to and didn't want to go to. At first blush it seemed like some simple but boring "cut and paste" homework.

But then I had an epiphany: why don't I plan this make-believe driving trip around visits to restaurants featured on Guy Fieri's *Diners, Drive-ins and Dives* TV show? If you haven't seen it, you're missing a piece of Americana. The host, Guy Fieri, is an awesome chef and a righteous dude. In his show he visits these terrific restaurants which serve food that us common folks can afford and love to eat, i.e. restaurants that make great barbeque sandwiches, monster pancakes or homemade corned beef hash.

I started out by plotting a route that had me driving four hundred and seventy nine miles from Chicagoland to *Big Momma's* restaurant in Omaha. *Big Momma's* signature dish was her sweet potato pie ice cream which sounded delicious. I then charted a five hundred mile trip to *Luxury Diner* in Cheyenne, Wyoming which had great reviews for its green chili on the *Yelp* website, and so on.

Planning the trip from diner to drive-in to dive was a blast, and probably exercised the old noggin' too. I had to figure out how far to drive each day, which *Diner, Drive-in or Dive* restaurant I wanted to eat at, and how to get there. I slapped the restaurants, directions and mileage onto some Excel spreadsheet.

At my next session, I quickly said "hi" to my savvy, model-thin, red-headed therapist as I marched in and plunked myself down at a desk in her teeny, tiny office full of eye charts, testing equipment and file drawers. I flipped open my laptop and explained that I needed it to show her my homework. Right away I could see that she not only liked the spreadsheets and schedules, but also thought Guy Fieri was a hoot.

And while she was happy, I was ecstatic. It was so nice to get positive feedback that I positively glowed for the rest of the day. And while I still haven't been to any of those restaurants, you can bet that if I ever get to Salt Lake City, I'm stopping at the Blue Plate Diner on 2100 East Street for some huevos rancheros verde.

While I battled rehab, Louis was fighting a losing battle with his health. The vet had ratcheted up his medication levels, which may have eased his pain but didn't make it any easier for him to walk. His left rear leg was so arthritic it barely touched the ground when he walked. We also had a hard time getting him in and out of the house. Since our first floor was actually a half story above ground level, he had to descend steps down to get to the back yard. If I tried to help him by holding up his arthritic legs, he'd turn his head to snap at me. This was something new. I loved my dog and the thought that he'd bite me hurt as much as if he'd actually bitten me.

Because he had so much trouble getting in and out of the house, I'd asked a friend to design a ramp that would let him walk down from one of our back doors, much like the wheel chair ramps for handicapped folks.

I felt like Louis and I were on divergent paths. I had finished my antibiotics and, according to my Lumosity scores, continued to climb out of the *Bottom 10%*. Louis seemed to be slowly stumbling down a one-way street that would end up someplace very bad.

Rehab, for me, was a lot like going to school in the third grade. I knew I had to do it. I knew I had to learn all that stuff. I just didn't like it all that much.

"Not liking something," though, was no excuse for avoiding rehab and it was a lot more important than anything I did in the third grade like flunk handwriting. Like most everybody I met in rehab, the temptation, irrational as it was, was to hang onto the past and tell myself "Hey, I've driven for 40 years, why do I have to do all this crap?"

The answer was pretty simple; because I've had a brain tumor. I'm not the same guy I'd been for the past 58 years and I might not be a safe driver. It was hard to admit, but it was the truth and, yes, at first I couldn't handle the truth.

At that time I felt that to succeed in rehab I had to have a positive attitude and be tenaciously determined. I believe that having a positive attitude is the most important. Being positive helped me make the effort to be tenacious. Losing that positive attitude just makes it a lot harder to diligently do my rehab exercises. Every time I started getting a negative attitude, rehab just became harder and easier to give up in favor of a book or a fun website.

And, try as I may, I still haven't found any book entitled "The Benefits of a Very Negative Mental Attitude", or "Negative Mental Attitudes can Definitely Improve Your Life!" or "Better Living through Negative Thinking."

For me, negative thinking was a trapdoor to dangerous "Why Me?" territory. Once I was trapped in "Why me-ness", I found myself slipping into the treacherous "Woe is me" waters of self-pity. The muck of self-pity was more quicksand than anything else and was really, really tough to climb out of by myself. So I tried really, really hard not to take one step down that path.

At the same time, I also learned that the rehab staff was not going to give me any pep talks or special motivation to tackle *my* problem. That's not their job. They knew how to assess my problems and assign exercises and programs to address them. It was my job to do the hard work, the rehab exercises.

To stay out of the emotional muck that was ever lurking, I tried to make the rehab as fun as possible, reward myself as often as possible and keep score so I could track my progress as closely as possible.

At the end of March, I ran out of insurance-paid rehab sessions and reached a plateau on Lumosity. I'd also passed my indoor rehab assessment and was approved for an over-the-road driving test which I couldn't wait to take. I felt like if I just took a few more "short choppy steps," I would be able to maximize my "new normal" and put this all behind me.

I saw these "short choppy steps" as passing my driver's test, having my cranioplasty (i.e. having my skull put back together) and going through radiation. In my mind, I needed to be as healthy as I could be to clear all three hurdles. After that, I'd be done. I would be able to drive myself. I would show up at work (if I got hired) without wearing a dorky blue helmet. I wouldn't have to ask for days off for radiation treatments. I would be normal.

I couldn't wait.

In my mind, April 26th was destined to be a turning point for me. At 1:30 in the afternoon my son would drive me to the rehab clinic where I would take my "over-the-road" driver's test. At 4:30 p.m. the same afternoon, Barbara and I would meet with *The Good Doctor* to talk about the endgame: completion surgery and radiation.

As Ernie Banks, the exuberant Chicago Cubs outfielder would say, "Let's play two!"

While winter was slowly loosening its death grip on the city, it was still cold. Personally, I think that spring is the cruelest month in Chicago. Why? You're dog-tired of snow and cold and you just plain crave a little, just a little sun and warmth. Instead, in the spring of 2011, we got an April that, according to the *Chicago Sun-Times* was the rainiest April on record, and it felt like it.

The rain made walking Louis, if you could call our turgid pace walking, a burden instead of a bracing bit of exercise.

On the day of the test, I felt strong. I felt confident; I felt ready. I'd been attending weight-training classes with a teacher that pushed me to my limit and slightly beyond. I'd been aggressively biking in spin classes to build new brain cells which I read about in Barbara Strauch's book, *The Secret Life of the Grown-Up Brain*. And I continued to work Lumosity, the HART chart and all the other eye exercises up to the last minute to make sure I was scanning through my blind spot and would "ace" my test.

My son drove me down to the rehab center where I was to meet the two judges: an impartial therapist (the ones who had worked with me were thought to be biased) and a driving evaluator. In the briefing literature, the center also stipulated that a family member or friend drive you down to the test. I liked that idea; I also wanted another pair of eyes and ears to see and hear the feedback from the test so I didn't fall into a "selective hearing" trap.

I felt pretty confident when I stepped into the car with a therapist and a driving instructor (my son stayed behind) for the all-important "over-the-road" test.

We started on nearly neighborhood roads with little traffic. My first comeuppance was being told that I needed to wait three seconds at every stop sign. I swallowed a "What? Nobody does that!" and tried to politely reply "thank you for the reminder" as other cars whizzed by with "rolling" stops.

Soon the grumpy driving instructor commented that I should cut holes in my blue helmet so I could better see. My initial reaction was one of confusion: didn't this mope know that this helmet had to pass through a bazillion committees full of persnickety doctors before it was approved for fragile patients with partial skulls? Did he think I bought this at K-Mart? Had he ever worked with somebody like me? Before I could reply, the therapist quickly said that she believed that I shouldn't and wouldn't be allowed to cut holes in the helmet by my neurosurgeon.

We continued down some more neighborhood streets before venturing out onto arterial roads with stop lights and two-way traffic. I felt strange looks being passed behind my back.

As I did so, the grumpy instructor commented that I wasn't exactly in the "middle" of my lane.

We then drove onto the highway, exited after a few miles and circled back to the center. They asked me to go wait for them in the foyer while they discussed my performance.

About five minutes later they came in and asked David and myself to join them in the conference room. The driving instructor decided not to sit down and, instead, stood up with his arms folded in a position of power and what seemed like confrontation.

They then recited their issues with my driving: starting to stop too early for some stop signs; not centering the car accurately in my lane; accelerating too quickly on the highway. They also thought that, with some on-the-road lessons, I might be able to drive. The implication, which was all too obvious, was that they thought I wasn't a safe driver.

That was hard to hear.

It was even harder to hear with my son sitting right next to me. Obviously Dad was handicapped or passed the threshold into codger-dom or both.

Damn.

Well, at least I would get the green light for surgery this afternoon.

As Barb and I drove to *The Good Doctor's* office, I was still in a funk from flunking my driver's test. In this country not being able to drive is tantamount to becoming a second class citizen, and given my fragile ego, I felt that I was barely second class. Moreover, I was embarrassed in front of my son. I could imagine what he was thinking, and I imagined that none of it was filed under the label of "good" or "pride" or "I want to be like him." The thought of taking more driving lessons from the grumpy instructor just made things worse. I felt like I was a drowning sailor and somebody had just thrown me an anchor.

The only thing that cheered me up was the thought of seeing *The Good Doctor* and literally getting my head together. I also expected the tumor to have shrunk because she told us that she'd cut off the blood supply to *The Blob* and, as a result, it should have shrunken significantly since the original operation.

But when Barbara and I arrived at *The Good Doctor's* office, after some initial polite conversation, she looked at my head and said:

> According to my recent Visual Field Test, my post-surgery vision was just about the same as my impaired pre-surgery vision. Okay, I could live with that.
>
> I had a scab on the back of my head from the drainage ditch. I suspected that the stapling technique had something to do with this, but didn't say so because I didn't want to sound like a whiner. Because of the scab, though, no surgery could start until that was completely healed. I was disappointed, but this not a deal-breaker for me.
>
> The latest MRI indicated that the tumor had not shrunk and, in fact, had started to, ever so slightly, grow again.

Wait a minute, this was a deal-breaker! This wasn't what I was expecting to hear. *The Blob* not only hasn't shrunk, it's on the comeback trail? Surgery is delayed? I felt sucker-punched and lower than whale snot.

The Good Doctor also made a quick, little, almost off-hand statement to the effect that, as I remember it, "radiation works in 95% of the cases." All the way home I wondered about her decision to say that. Did she suspect I was a "five percenter?" Did she smell an unhappy ending? What would happen if the Blob grew back? Another surgery? More radiation? A dip back into the *Bottom 10%*?

I had no smart-alecky comment, no "bon-mots," and no quick quips. Somehow I felt like my rehab effort, my good soldiering was all wasted. I was wasting time on the fruitless thought that I could win this war or even negotiate a face-saving peace. I was feeling the pain and not liking it one little bit.

A little voice in the back of my head suggested that maybe I just ought to take a long swim off the short and nearby Gilson Park pier on Lake Michigan.

While I sort of knew it, I was being sucked into dangerous psychological waters way over my head. I found myself recounting the facts that I had no job, no prospects of a job and no idea of anybody who would hire me. And, in our family, being jobless was just about one of the worst sins somebody could commit. I just felt like a useless boob of a husband, a non-contributing father and a drag on the family finances. The idea of jumping in Lake Michigan and swimming east towards the State of Michigan started to sound more and more like a real option.

A few days later I tried to change my attitude by changing my environment and attending a crowded industry function in downtown Chicago. Given the train schedule, I arrived early and grabbed a seat at a nearby coffee shop. As I waited, I once again, felt that the only way I could express my feelings was through lyrics (sung to the tune of "Run Around Sue"):

> Here's my story, it's sad but true
> It's about my tumor making me blue
> It took my health and ran around
> Breakin' all the synapses in town
>
> Whoa…whoa…(sing this a lot)
>
> Ah, I should have known it from the very first date
> This disease will infect my bone plate
> Now listen people what I'm telling you
> I've got a case of *Brain Tumor Blues*

More whoa-ing

I miss the power of my clear thinking brain
With this tumor I'll never be the same
So if you don't wanna pine like I do
Keep away from Brain Tumor Blues

Ah, Blob likes to spread it around
And he'll drag your eyesight down
Now people let me put you wise
He's ooouut to squish your little eyes

Here's the moral of the story from a guy who knows
I have tumor and the tumor still grows
Ask any fool that the Blob ever knew, they'll say
Keep away from the Brain Tumor Blues

Whoa…woe…woe (repeat a lot)

I read this to Barbara over the phone. She suggested that I keep this one to myself.

The Good Wife:

"Johnny and Barbie in a tree
K-i-s-s-i-n-g.
First comes love, then they're wed,
Then comes Johnny in a doctor's bed."

About this time, folks would call me up, get an update on my health and quickly ask "How's Barbara doing?" Well, it's probably time for her performance review, so here's my first draft. On the plus side she:

Endured my first stay in the hospital.
Continued her stellar work performance in spite of my health woes.
Went to the hospital each day during my second trip of eleven days.

Tried to sleep during our fun with the French Male Purse.
Cut my hair including the part which covered my missing scalp.
Handled a ton of complicated medical bills and forms.
And did a bunch of other stuff I forgot.

On the "need for improvement" side, ummm, well, I can't think of anything other than she sometimes steals the blanket on cold nights.

Here's my self-evaluation for the time period covering our first learning about *The Blob*. On the negative side, I:

Had a little disagreement with nurse "don't-bother-me."
Landed in the bottom 10%.
Took eleven days to complete a three day medication assignment.
Woke Barbara up a 7 a.m. every day for six weeks to give me a "fix."
Had to be driven everywhere beyond walking distance of the mass transit system.
Was a significant drain on the family budget.
And did a bunch of other stuff I've tried to forget.

On the plus side, I don't think I stole the down comforter even once.

6

The Gun Lap

IN SPITE OF WORRIES ABOUT *THE BLOB,* and a delayed schedule for my cranioplasty and radiation treatments, in early May I felt like I was entering the final phase of my journey. Having run track in high school, I vividly remembered the sharp gunshot which announced to all runners that they were starting the final lap of the race. In early May I had that same feeling: that while I had a few more, pretty high hurdles to jump, the end of this part of my journey was within reach.

This "gun lap" feeling was heightened by the fact that I was actually running to get in shape for the American Brain Tumor Association's *Pathway to Progress* five kilometer fun run. I read that the funds were being raised for brain tumor research, so I decided to sign up and give something back to the brain tumor community.

The morning of the fun run, the weather was downright unfriendly: gusty and cold. Nonetheless, Barb and I got our butts out of bed and zipped downtown at an unusually early hour for a weekend morning. The fun run began right next to the Soldier Field football stadium alongside the lake. The whole area felt like an extension of the museum campus which included the Adler Planetarium, the Field Museum and the Shedd Aquarium. Instead of feeling like the epicenter of the city, the venue felt more like a big park. It was a great place for a fun run.

I'm not sure what I was expecting for a turnout. If you'd asked me, I might have guessed upwards of a couple of hundred runners and, given the cool temperature and stiff breeze, a few friends and family members.

I was wrong.

Thousands of people were there: friends, families, kids in strollers, kids who should have been in strollers, runners, walkers, folks who needed walkers, survivors, victims, victims in wheel chairs and at least one victim wearing a dorky blue helmet (no, that wasn't me, I ran without my helmet… and please don't tell the lady from the infectious disease department).

Everybody seemed to be wearing a motivational shirt of some sort. A lot of people were wearing the official dark purple *Pathway to Progress* t-shirt, but many were wearing brightly-colored, custom-designed team t-shirts. They had names like "Madeline's Milers," "Legs for Lin," "Go for Joe," and my favorite team name, "Tommie's Tumors."

I had found my "peeps'." I had found a community of folks who, like me, were battling a nasty, unfair and relentless enemy. Unlike me, they were doing so with faith, strength and a touch of panache. I walked around the staging area with a goofy smile on my face. Of course, I also felt that way at Michigan State University football games when everybody wears a Spartan t-shirt, so I guess I'm easily swayed by a crowd.

When the gun went off to start the race, I couldn't wait to run. There was something fundamentally inspirational about running with this group. So I ran, enjoyed the lake view, shouted encouragement to other runners and had a blast. And in spite of the high-tech timing device that I wore on my wrist, I had no idea what my time was and I didn't care.

After the race Barbara and I hung around oblivious to the cold and windy weather. We looked at the lake, grabbed a cup of nearly hot coffee and enjoyed being part of the crowd. As we strolled, we talked about how next year we'd recruit our own team, get our own t-shirt design, get our own team name, and have a group of walkers and runners. Even though we didn't say it, I knew then we would really, truly be part of the community.

In addition to training for the fun run, I tried to take as many driving lessons as I could with my new best friend, the grumpy driving instructor. We would start on thinly traveled neighborhood streets which, come warmer weather, would be lined with thick green lawns and tall leafy trees. After that "warm-up," he'd ask me to venture onto more crowded streets with two-way traffic, Northwestern University students dashing between cars and honest-to-goodness traffic lights. If I seemed ready, we'd veer over towards the expressway and we'd get to see if I could merge into traffic. For a few brief seconds, I'd accelerate up to fifty-five miles an hour before exiting for a debrief. In every lesson, we took this mid-lesson break and he told me what

I did wrong and what I needed to do to correct those mistakes. I never, ever remember him saying "good job" or "keep that up" or "I like what you're doing".

Maybe they taught him in instructor training school that positive feedback was a sign of weakness. Or maybe he just never, ever thought I did anything right (which was certainly possible). In either case, I found the sessions to be particularly disheartening and demoralizing. Barbara would come home frustrated from a tough day at the office, ask me about my training and become even more frustrated. I didn't want to upset her so, after a while, stopped telling her about it.

I also continued to work on my visual scanning and "spatial relations" skills. After a few more weeks, the weather finally woke up, realized it was spring, and the sun started to shine a bit. Since this was Chicagoland, it was still too cold to walk around in sandals, a pair of shorts and a Hawaiian shirt. I know because I tried and nearly froze. Louis, even in his gimpy condition, still never seemed to be bothered by the weather be it hot, cold, snowing or, during some walks, raining.

In addition to being cosmically linked to Louis, for months I also felt oddly linked to Gabby Giffords. I remember hearing the news of her shooting in early January and being horrified. The following news article stated the facts:

> On January 8, 2011, Giffords was a victim of a shooting near Tucson, which was reported to be an assassination attempt on her, at a Safeway supermarket where she was meeting publicly with constituents. Giffords was critically injured by a gunshot wound to the head; six people were killed, among them conservative federal judge John Roll, who had received death threats two years earlier. Another thirteen people were injured in the shooting.[2]

Shortly after that, it was widely reported that she had surgery to remove portions of her skull to accommodate the ensuing swelling. Well I knew what that was all about; I also had a portion of my skull removed, albeit for a different reason. For me, the news was a sober reminder that, no matter how bad you think you have it, somebody always has it worse. I can't say that it made me feel better, but it did remind me that my recovery point was starting from a higher ridge on the rehab mountain.

In mid-May I read the following:

> Gabrielle Giffords is recovering after surgery to repair her skull. On Wednesday doctors put a plastic implant in place to cover her brain, according to a statement from TIRR Memorial Hermann hospital in Houston.[3]

It was in all the papers and on all the news channels. In an eerie way our paths were progressing quite similarly. The news also gave me a way to describe my next surgery so that others could understand it, i.e. "I'm having the Gabby Giffords surgery."

In many ways she was an excellent role model; a traumatic brain injury victim who, as far as I knew, didn't complain, didn't quit and expected to return to her job. And if that wasn't true, that's what her staff led me to believe. So I tried to mimic her "never say die" attitude. (Okay, maybe that's a poor choice of words. How about her tenacious, "can do" attitude?)

Just about the time I read about Gabby's surgery, my drainage ditch scab healed and *The Good Doctor* pronounced me fit for my cranioplasty.

I expected her to reinsert my old skull having been disinfected by the super deep freezer in which it had been stored for the past several months. I had this mental picture of a large white Kenmore chest freezer stashed in some obscure and dimly lit basement room of the hospital. I had friends who had separate freezers, and it seemed that they were constantly sorting through a pile of frozen items in zip-locked bags that had lost their labels. I have this memory of one friend trying to figure out if he was holding a pound of ground chuck or a pound of meatloaf mix and still not being sure after he opened it.

The thought of *The Good Doctor*, in her stylish attire, taking the elevator down to the sub-basement, opening up the freezer and pawing through a variety of frozen body parts to find mine, brought a smile to my face.

Of course that's just being silly. Being a high-class, twenty-first century hospital, I'm sure that they have a large walk-in freezer with various steel bins so that the frozen skulls aren't thrown in with the, gee I don't know, all the other bones and organs they freeze and reuse.

No matter where *The Good Doctor* stored my skull, I believe that she or her assistant told me that they let it gently defrost[t] (no microwaving that I know of) to see if the dangerous, slow-growing, non-oxygen-based bacterial infection had been killed. After being defrosted, though, the bacteria started to sprout just like the weeds in my lawn following our long, cold winter. So we went to plan "B" which included replacing my resected rear bone plate, i.e. the back of my skull, with a sanitized, freshly-minted plastic job.

At first I was a bit worried about not getting my original piece of skull back. But my tall, lanky son said, "After all the trouble that old skull gave you, do you really want it back?" It was a good point. So I decided that a prosthetic skull would do just fine.

One of *The Good Doctor's* vigilant assistants made sure that all the appropriate paperwork was filled out prior to my cranioplasty, i.e. prosthetic replacement. So it wasn't really a surprise when I received a note from the insurance company telling me that they would cover the cost of the operation. The wording of the letter, however, was a bit off-putting.

Your health benefits plan requires some services to be reviewed for approval. We received a coverage request on 05/12/2011 for you for the following services(s):
Approved: Repair Skull Defect

Now, when somebody says "This part was defective," what do you think? I think that means the part was "defective" from the moment it rolled off of the manufacturing line. In Detroit-speak, I was a "Friday baby", i.e. the day that many seasoned veterans call in sick and the cars get made by substitute workers with experience and skills that result in a car of less than top quality. To my way of thinking, the note implied that my skull, and maybe my entire head, was flawed from the "get go." It's an "A-HA" moment that raised some serious questions. For example, if my skull was *always* defective:

"How did I get into Michigan State University?" (If you're a Wolverine, don't answer that.)
"How come my head didn't just crack open like an egg when I played football in the eighth grade?" (On the other hand, at 135 lbs. soaking wet, I just bounced off of everybody anyways.)

"How would you know?" Was there some sort of genetic testing that could verify this?"

Now I know what you're thinking, "Did you check the warranty?" Well, smarty-pants, I tried. I called up my Mom and Dad and asked them point-blank: "Did you get a warranty when you had me?" Their answer wasn't entirely satisfactory. They hemmed and hawed and then said something like, "John, you know that we were quite poor back then."

About that time I reread another pre-cranioplasty surgery report from *The Good Doctor*. In the report, there was a line that said: "Patient denies double vision, blurry vision, weakness, or numbness".

Now, I had been on some heavy drugs ("Man") following the operation. So I don't remember a conversation with a doctor in which I denied all these accusations, but I can imagine it going something like this:

"Mr. Kerastas, do you deny that you have double vision?"
"Yes."
"Do you deny having blurry vision?"
"Yes."
"Do you deny weakness?"
"Yes."
"Do you deny numbness?"
"Yes."
"Do you deny being in the *Bottom 10%*?"
"No."
"I rest my case."

Just prior to the surgery I got a lot of questions from friends and family, most of which included the word "how." How would they determine whether to just patch the hole in your skull or glue in a prosthetic substitute? If they just patch the hole, how do they do that? How do you know the patch will stay in place? Is it like a shingle roof that you have to replace every fifteen years or so? Will it leak if you don't replace it before the warranty runs out?

These questions were somewhat primed by Pastor Jane's announcement, to the entire congregation, that "John is going to get the hole in his head fixed this week." And, yes, she giggled when she said it.

I soon learned that with small head holes, the operation is a lot like dry walling. Your surgeon puts a bit of netting over the hole and then spreads something pretty similar to plaster of Paris over the netting until the hole is filled or plaster starts leaking out your nose.

If you have an extra-large head hole (that phrase somehow makes it sounds like you're a whale) the surgeon will order a pre-fabricated blow-hole piece that comes in the usual men's and women's sizes: small, medium, large, and politician.

You might ask, "Are these prosthetic skull pieces always bought in standard off-the-shelf sizes or can you get a custom-built job?"

The answer depends upon:

A. Your insurance plan.
B. You socio-economic circumstances.
C. Your life expectancy.
D. What your wife orders.

The correct answer, as you should know by now, is "D."

The last question most folks asked prior to the surgery was: "What do they make prosthetic skulls out of?" The answer, and I'm not making this up[5], is basically the same hard, durable plastic that is used to make bowling balls. I am also hoping it will make it a lot easier to roll with the hard knocks I seem to keep having.

I was told that one of the advantages to using the porous bowling ball-like material is that bone cells will, over time, float into the prosthetic insert and better seal the deal. In preparing for the operation *The Good Doctor* had two prosthetic inserts made for the operation should one, I guess, slip out of somebody's hands, bounce on the floor and get dirty. The prosthetic itself was sort of a bone-like translucent whitish color which is good because I didn't want to get into a color argument with my wife, e.g. "You're a 'winter' and should consider a deep grey or maybe even a black prosthetic to contrast with the rest of your skull."

When I first saw it, it seemed rather thin which made me wonder if it was all that strong? Of course, how can you tell? Whack it with a hammer a few times and if it doesn't break say, "looks good to me?"

Prior to the operation I also had to have a "staph infection" test. I wasn't sure what this all meant, so I looked it up on Medicine.net where I found out that:

MRSA is a type of Staphylococcus aureus (S. aureus). Staphylococcus aureus, often referred to simply as 'staph', are bacteria commonly carried on the skin or in the nose of healthy people.

My first thought was, "what's the big deal?" I then read that:

MRSA infections are usually mild, superficial infections of the skin that can be treated successfully with proper skin care and antibiotics. MRSA, however, can be difficult to treat and **can progress to life-threatening blood or bone infections** because there are fewer effective antibiotics available for treatment (bold emphasis added).

A bit further down the page I learned that "MRSA infections occur commonly among persons in hospitals and healthcare facilities."

Hmmm, let me see. I have a history of getting bone infections during operations, and most staph infections, which are really bad, happen in hospitals. Yes, we needed to find out if I had a staph infection. So I had a pre-op test and found out that, yes indeed, I had a staph infection.

There is a lot of misinformation about staph, so I thought it would be helpful if I shared what I learned with you in the form of a "Question and Answer" format.

Question: "Were you informed that you had a staph infection?"
Answer: "No. I was informed that I had staph 'colonies.' Colonies are merely precursors to a full-scale infection and, as a result, aren't anything to be completely panicked about. I was only half-panicked when told about the colonies."
Question: "Which half?"
Answer: "The top half. Most of my problems come from the top of my head."

Question: "So what did you do about it?"

Answer: "The correct procedure is to stick (no, not that kind of 'stick') a swab up your nose with powerful ointment on it to kill, as possible, the colonies."

Question: "How did you feel about that?"

Answer: "I felt like I was back in the third grade sticking things in places they don't belong."

Question: "Did it work?"

Answer: "I haven't noticed any 'staph' meetings or agendas in my nose, but then again it's hard to see given my long thick nose hairs."

My operation was scheduled for the end of May. Chicagoland was finally shaking off the lingering coldness as the sun was shining more than it rained, and temperatures warmed up. The record rains led to grassy lawns, thick leaves and a record numbers of flies, mosquitos and flying critters.

Barbara and all our children rode along with me to the hospital. Since this wasn't like the first operation for a fist-sized tumor or an emergency visit for a dangerous infection, everybody felt a lot more relaxed, including me.

Up to now I knew one thing about hospitals; I was pretty good at checking in and pretty lousy at checking out. This time, however, *The Good Doctor* was all over my schedule like hair on a bear.

What did that mean? It meant that the fix was in. It meant that everybody—the residents, the nurses and even the food service staff—all knew that I was scheduled to get in and get out in forty-eight hours.

And I did.

As usual, I checked in early and was escorted to a staging room. I seem to remember having a late morning operation as the sun was already reasonably high in the sky when the orderly came to fetch me.

The one little speed bump in the entire procedure happened the first night. After I asked to be escorted to the lavatory at 1 a.m., 2 a.m. and 3 a.m., a large, fleshy male nurse decided that I needed to be catheterized. The thought of being catheterized just brought back all sorts of bad memories about strange malfunctioning microcomputers and the wrong antibiotics from earlier in the year. In spite of my visible shivering, he left to get some special instrument to help him decide. I started to imagine the kind of instrument he needed to help decide if I needed to be catheterized, and everything I imagined seemed left over from the Spanish Inquisition.

He brought back an oddly-shaped, high-tech wand which he waved over my lower abdomen. The wand was, thankfully, a non-invasive bladder tank detector. In my case, I had a full tank. So, he strode off to go talk to the resident about it.

The idea of getting my, err, private parts catheterized brought back the willies in full force. I didn't like the idea. I didn't want to like the idea. I wasn't going to like the idea.

I imagined one of my healthier buddies saying something like "I hear that term, 'catheterized' used all the time, what does it really mean?" How would I answer that? "Well they take a drinking straw, no not the ones they use for bubble tea, and stick it up the downspout."

I couldn't imagine anybody talking about it as a rite of passage or as some male bravado as in "I was hoping you'd catheterize me—now I can tell all the guys!" or "Yah, it's time to let the air out of my balloon"; or even "Since my ego's in the *Bottom 10%*, let's deflate my bladder, too."

Of course, I'm just guessing. So why don't you conduct a little survey among your closest male friends. The following multiple choice quiz (chose one) will do just fine:

A. I think being catheterized will be a mind expanding experience, go ahead.
B. I have it on my bucket list.
C. Well, now that you mention it, I am feeling a bit clogged myself.
D. Come near me and I'll shoot!

If you don't know the answer by now, I'm not going to tell you.

In the end, he wound up catheterizing me. While it hurt physically, it hurt a lot more psychologically. And, if he smirked, at least he had the common decency to do it behind my back.

Luckily, the day shift was filled with nurses I knew and liked from previous stays. When I wasn't sleeping they came into my room, chatted, laughed and, in general, made the stay bearable.

The following morning it was clear that *The Good Doctor's* Chicago-style fix was in. I was expelled shortly before lunch, a new land speed record.

My recovery from the cranioplasty was reasonably smooth and I was now focused on passing my driver's test, preparing for my radiation treatments and managing a pro bono project for a terrific non-profit organization. As it turned out, I was scheduled to take my driver's test the afternoon of my first presentation to the board of the non-profit's board of directors.

The day before the test and presentation, though, was the toughest day in this long, drawn-out, seemingly endless race to recovery, and it started with Louis. In the morning I was able to get him out of the house and into the back yard. He had a hard time getting his head down to his stainless steel food dish, so I held it up to his mouth for him to eat. That afternoon though, Louis, our once-proud, raccoon-fighting, shot-from-a-gun fast dog, was so weak and arthritic he couldn't even get up off the ground from a nap.

I'd been expecting and dreading this moment. For months, his downward spiral, and my health issues, seemed to be cosmically linked. We both went from bad to worse during the long, bitterly cold Chicago winter.

At some point, though, and for reasons that I can't quite grasp, our paths diverged. Even with antibiotic missteps, a catheterized left-arm and rehab hurdles, I've gotten healthier and even had a whole head. I could now sleep nearly eight hours, my Lumosity scores were improving and even my self-image was marginally better.

I watched him as he floundered on his right side and struggled to get up. His two front legs had some strength, but his rear legs were so arthritic he could barely put any weight on them. When I tried to help him stand up by lifting his arthritic legs, he snapped at me. The snapping told me that, in spite of the meds I'd given him, he was in incredible pain. I tried to calm him down by rubbing him in his favorite spot under his jaw and feeding him water from my hands, but it didn't seem to help.

So he spent a lot of time trying to get up, failing. And, during all this, he's yelping with pain. His yelping is so bad, I'm surprised the neighbors don't come over to see what's wrong.

I yearned to take him to the vet, but I was home alone, and didn't have a car.

One of the ironies of that day was that it was absolutely beautiful outside. The sun was shining, the temperature was warm, flies were buzzing gently and my dog was dying a painful death.

At the time I couldn't help thinking, "Is this some crazy foreshadowing of my own demise? Will I be writhing in pain, or just juiced with so much pain killer that even I won't know when I die?" Even now, years later, I think of my mother-in-law's death and the agonizing decision my wife, sister-in-laws and brother-in-law faced when they turned off her life support. Nothing about these decisions seem easy, they all seem fraught with second-guessing and "what ifs?"

Barbara couldn't get home until after our vet closed. So after she got home, we scooted Louis onto a beach blanket and carried him in the back door and onto the mudroom floor to make him comfortable (and keep the bugs away from him). We packed the room with pillows so he wouldn't bang into the wooden steps or tiles as he thrashed. Then, we took turns that night sitting with him, feeding him, giving him water and giving him pain-killers until our vet opened the next morning. Our youngest daughter, for whom we originally bought the dog, drove up from the city and helped us take him to the vet. She was with us when we put our beautiful, blond-haired part German shepherd, part Labrador down. We had him cremated and, one day, I plan to take his ashes and scatter them on the dog beach as the days running with all the other dogs were probably some of the happiest days of his life.

I think we got back home around 11 a.m. My wife and Jenny were needed at work, so they reluctantly climbed into their cars and drove off.

And while I wanted to take a quick nap before my 1 p.m. driver's test, the raw emotions of the previous night and morning just whirled around and around in my head. So after twenty minutes or so, I showered and hopped a suburban bus to the "El" stop (i.e. electric train station) for a ride to meet my grumpy driving instructor and my therapist for my driving test. This was, of course, one of my dumber decisions as I was emotionally wrung out and dead tired.

The skill set and acumen I needed to demonstrate was more stringent than for a normal driver of my age because I had a brain tumor and was partially blind. When I first learned of this from one of my therapists, I was pissed off, especially when I saw all the yahoos (i.e. other drivers) on the road that ignored neighborhood stop signs, checked email while driving and forgot that their cars did indeed have turn signals.

While my main therapist wasn't schedule for the evaluation, due to possible biases, the alternate therapist was a sharp and personable lady whom I'd worked with a few times. She had dark curly hair, empathetic eyes that didn't miss a thing and a wonderfully warm smile. I told her about being up for over the past twenty-four hours and she smartly asked me if I still wanted to have the test. In spite of the strain from Louis' death, I dumbly answered "yes."

In spite of her obvious misapprehensions, she said, "Okay." She was also training a new therapist and asked if she could come along for the ride. I said "sure" and probably something flip like, "The more the merrier."

The test started out bad and got worse. We rode through the same quiet neighborhoods with nice green lawns and tall trees that I'd done during my training. But I was so tired that I felt that I was driving through totally unknown territory. My reflexes just seemed not one, but two beats slow. And while I didn't feel that I was dangerous, I knew that I wasn't meeting the higher standards I had met in my previous training sessions. It was an unsettling feeling. I thought I could do this and couldn't. All my life I had succeeded at almost everything I tackled. I got good grades in high school and college. I got promotions at my first employer. I felt that I really helped the start-up companies I'd worked at. But at the halfway mark of the test, where we always stopped so they could give me an interim assessment, I knew I was failing and told them so.

Somehow, Mr. Grumpy talked me into finishing the ride so I forced myself back into the driver's seat of his specially equipped car (the car was outfitted so he could wrest control of it from me at a moment's notice if needed) and finished the test.

When we got back to the facility, they asked me to sit in the waiting room while they talked and discussed my performance. The rehab waiting room was one of my least favorite places to wait. The room was small and always seemed crowded. The aseptic wooden chairs with worn-out plastic cushions were just plain uncomfortable. And the receptionist always seemed to be on the phone trying to straighten out some scheduling snafu that the person on the other end was upset about.

I waited and waited. I started to worry about getting to my non-profit meeting on time as I needed to catch the El transfer at the Howard Street station and ride down to the Uptown area in the city proper for my meeting.

I wasn't sure how often the trains ran at that time of day, but I really didn't want to get there late.

As I waited, I couldn't figure out what the problem was. I knew I didn't pass. They knew I didn't pass. What were they doing in there, playing pinochle? Finally, they called me into her tiny office. I felt like all four of us were crammed into a really old elevator or one of those Japanese hotel rooms were you can't even stand up straight. The senior therapist sat down and asked me to sit across from her. The therapist-in-training sat to my far right. Mr. Grumpy stood up between the two of them, crossed his arms, stuck out his belly and looked ready for a fight.

Strangely, the senior therapist started out by asking me how I felt I did. I answered something to the effect that what difference would that make? She then said that it was really important. I was confused, why would that matter? Nonetheless I tried to simply, and as unemotionally as possible, state that I didn't pass. Those were hard words to say because they just reinforced all the self-doubts that were poised to drown my fragile self-confidence.

She then gave me her detailed assessment of the faults in my driving, and there were a lot. Here comments were accurate and to the point. Nonetheless, it still hurt to hear them.

The room seemed to becoming smaller, hotter and devoid of anything passing for fresh air. I felt like I was being interrogated in some 1930s police station as a homicide suspect instead of being debriefed on a driver's test. I sat next to one of the bulky machines that tested your reflex reactions, and it looked like it was designed in the 1940s and they bought it in the 1950s which reinforced that sensation. I was hoping that my reflexes and self-control were under control because Mr. Grumpy, who I could have also nicknamed "Mr. Negative," was next in line to speak.

He tightened his grip on his arms, looked down his nose at me and then began to recite, from the beginning, his recollection of my mistakes. As I watched him I thought that he must have been one of those ex-army drill instructors that everybody hated. I had this crazy impulse to say "Thank you sir, I'll have another," the phrase you were taught to say when you got paddled in junior high (yes, I went to junior high school in the dark ages). He added nothing new, and certainly nothing that would help me do better in the future, but I kept trying to nod "yes" so I could get this disaster over with as quickly as possible.

I was tired. I was disappointed and I was trying to find a way to politely leave because sneak peeks at my watch told me that I needed to catch the El pretty soon to make my non-profit meeting.

Then, all of a sudden the junior therapist began her synopsis. I thought of her as "Little Miss Suck-up" because she wanted the other two to know that she really, really agreed with them. She then started to talk as if I was more of a specimen than a person, and certainly a person that wasn't in the room. She reiterated my faults in, if it was possible, even greater detail than Mr. Grumpy. During her soliloquy I have almost no memory of her looking at me. I wasn't her audience. Her audience was the senior therapist and Mr. Grumpy. I hadn't felt like such a piece of meat since I'd had my vein catheterized. I didn't like it. I wasn't gonna like it. And I couldn't wait to get done with it.

Immensely proud of herself, she finally wrapped up her assertions like a first-rate criminal prosecutor. And, as much as I wanted to give her a fifteen yard penalty for piling on, I wasn't wearing a black and white striped referee shirt and was positive none of them would understand the relevant hand signals (and I tried very, very hard to avoid any other kind of hand signal).

The senior therapist then commented that they didn't want to see me for another three months, because maybe by then my tumor would shrink some more and I'd be more normal or capable or close to being human-like. My knee-jerk reaction was to say I never wanted to see any of them for the rest of my life, and I wasn't all that sure about them being human either. But, I swallowed those words and tried to take the high ground in my parting comments. Instead I think they were closer to Jim Carey's parting line in *The Truman Show* where he said, "Good morning. And in case I don't see you: good afternoon, good evening and good night."

I grabbed my black polyester mesh briefcase, hurried out the door and bolted down the street to the El stop. As I passed through the gates and onto the platform I reviewed the day. Let me see, my dog died a crappy death. I just flunked a driver's test. I was dead tired. I wanted to make a great impression to the non-profit board, but the odds didn't seem real good.

The non-profit's board meeting was taking place in an old building which was fighting benign neglect and an inadequate maintenance budget. The first floor meeting room was surprisingly large with a fifteen foot ceiling that gave a glimpse of past importance. As I gently peeked into the room, I saw at least twenty-five people seated around the center table, maybe more. This seemed to be a community that had an emotional connection to their organization and made a point to come to their meetings, instead of finding last-minute "emergencies" that, sadly, prevented their attendance.

Against a back wall was a delicious-smelling buffet as the meeting was held during dinner-time. Instead of checking out the executives seated around the room, I instinctively checked out the buffet: samosas, curries, nan, salad and several other interesting-looking dishes in stainless steel buffet containers. The fragrances were intoxicating. I thought I smelled some pungent chutney in there, too. Since I hadn't had anything to eat all day, my stomach started doing flip flops and making odd noises which I tried to ignore and hoped others couldn't hear.

The meeting was already in progress when I arrived. So I tried to pick my way over to an empty seat in the far back corner of the room and didn't stumble over more than two or three pairs of feet.

The classy and imperturbable Executive Director, though, saw me nearly trip and took that moment to introduce me to everybody in the room. I gave an embarrassed half wave much like Queen Elizabeth, and promptly sat down.

The non-profit had started as a battered women's shelter and had matured into a well-run agency providing a full range of services to immigrant communities. The board, like the buffet, was South Asian and given my Asian work experiences a nice fit for both of us. These were good people doing important work, and I was working on no sleep for the past thirty-six hours. I smelled a disaster in the making and thought that rather than try to be quick or witty or particularly articulate, I would make the shortest possible presentation and try to escape with what remained of my dignity.

Maybe fifteen minutes later there was a break and I had a chance to cue up the slide presentation. I told the Executive Director that I wouldn't belabor any of the points in my presentation. Actually, I had hoped that they were running hopelessly late so I could just give the "cliff notes" version. She told me, however, that they were on schedule and eager to hear about the services we would provide. So when everybody sat down, I stood up and started speaking.

I first caught on to the fact that I was talking too fast when the Executive Director smoothly clarified a point I was making. One slide later she did it again. I tried to zip through the next three slides, and she, without missing a beat, toggled back to the original slide and explained the points in the slide in greater detail to the slightly confused audience. I looked at the scrunched-up faces with tilting eyebrows and saw that it wasn't until she embellished my charts, and put the points in context, that they had any idea what I was talking about. My memory isn't all that clear, but I think right about then I sat down and let her give most of the rest of the presentation. While it wasn't a disaster of titanic proportions, it sure felt like I hadn't made that all-important good first impression.

Rats.

On the El on the way home I tried to forget the failures of the day and couldn't. I got home, threw my clothes in our large straw dirty-closes hamper and threw myself under the covers. Even though I was exhausted, I played the "what if" mind game for hours, like what if I said "no thank you" to taking the driver's test after staying up all night? I second-guessed myself into the wee hours of the morning.

Shortly thereafter I was scheduled for my radiation blast. I say blast, because *The Good Doctor*, in consultation with the radiologist, decided that instead of five days of radiation, I should have one blast of five days' worth of radiation. As I understood it, the five-in-one-blast had a better track record of preventing reoccurring tumor growth.

As soon as I heard this, I immediately thought of the original Uncle Fester from the *Adams Family* TV show. If you haven't seen it, Uncle Fester could turn on a light bulb just by popping it into his mouth. Don't think about it too much, it's a sight gag.

I tried not to think about the radiation and then, on a fine summer morning, Barbara hustled my lazy butt over to the hospital for my radiation mask fitting.

In order to make sure that only *The Blob* was radiated and not, for example, my ability to play the trombone or killer beer pong, I needed to hold my head very, very still during the treatment. Since radiologists stay up nights worrying about things like sneezing during beaming, the remedy is to custom-build a face mask that will keep your head in a locked down position and as still as possible. So a week or so prior to my radiation blast, I went to the hospital and had a warm, pliable white plastic mesh form molded to my face.

The resulting face mask had six pre-drilled holes in it so that the technicians could, literally, bolt me down to the table to keep me from moving, fidgeting or picking my nose.

As soon as I put the mask on, I thought I looked like Anthony Hopkins from the movie, *Silence of the Lambs*. I wanted to wear the mask on Halloween because I thought it would scare the snot out of kids who were trick or treating. Barbara, of course, said "you can't wear that; you'll scare the snot out of little kids." So I didn't.

The morning of the radiation blast the North Shore weather was wonderful and happy. The temperature was warm without being hot. Bees were harvesting pollen from flowers that seemed to be everywhere: in gardens, under bushes and in your lawns if you hadn't put down anti-dandelion spray.

While I felt like I'd been in almost every section of the hospital, I hadn't been in the radiation center.

When I first walked into the radiation theater, I saw a pleasant, serene little garden planted over by a large window. I suspect its job was to put me at ease and to help me think happy thoughts. Of course, a few steps later, I turned a corner and saw the radiation bed and the high-tech gamma-ray weaponry.

I then climbed onto the radiation bed and a technician bolted my head to my custom-molded mask. As I looked at the mask, I was slightly confused by the arrows drawn on the mask that clearly pointed out which holes were for the jaw and which were designed for the forehead. I couldn't imagine how somebody could bolt the mask on upside down, but could imagine what a disaster it would be if they did.

The "arms" of the five gamma-ray guns were attached to the ceiling equidistance from each other. I think the idea was that no one gamma ray beam would harm you (much) as they passed through your brain. They would all converge, though, from five points of the compass on aspects of *The Blob* and blast it into submission, or at least remission. And, since *The Blob* was in various parts of my brain, the blasters would be repositioned several times.

The gamma ray guns vaguely reminded me of the medical equipment from the movie *Alien*: futuristically sleek, spotlessly clean and antiseptically sterile. When they sprang into action and noiselessly repositioned themselves, I felt like I was being examined by some strangely observant alien life force that was saying to itself, "Hmmm, if I blast this bit here, I wonder if he'll walk like a turkey."

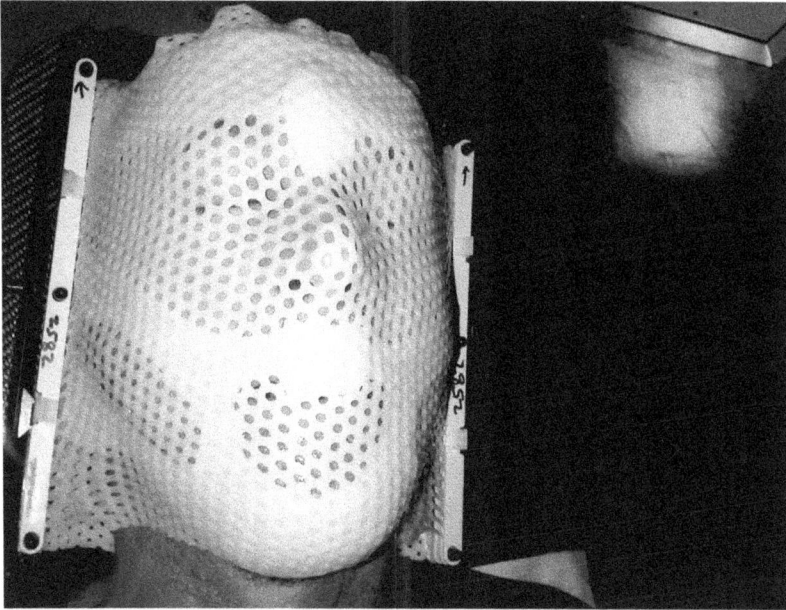

Barbara took this picture just before I got my radiation blast.

Like most things in life, the preamble to the radiation was scarier than the actual treatment. It didn't take that long and it didn't hurt[6].

Barbara and I walked out of the hospital and everything seemed the same. The sun shined, breezes blew and crows squawked. But I had changed. I was as newly normalized as I could be. It felt good.

I used to think that rehab and recovery was more like a marathon than a sprint because it was awfully long and hard, but I was wrong. It's more like steeple chase than a marathon. Why? Because even though it's long, every so often you have to jump a hurdle. It might be a cognitive hurdle, a physical hurdle or an emotional hurdle. Or all three, like a driver's test. Sometimes you clear the hurdle, and sometimes you fall on your face in the mud. That's no reason, though, to give up. You have to get up, wipe the mud off your face and get back in the race.

I'm done wiping, but I'm not done racing.

Epilogue

WHAT I DIDN'T EXPECT DURING THIS FIRST YEAR of "tumor time" was the emotional ups and downs I would encounter. Looking back on it, I can see that I avoided "feeling the pain" as much as possible. The four stages of emotional responses to a (natural) disaster that I learned about from the UMOR 2012 Disaster Response Academy are still the best description I've found of the emotions I experienced. During my emotional recovery I became a master at denial, at refusing to accept the reality of my situation. I joked, guffawed and made fun of my disease and handicaps sixteen-ways-from-Sunday. The worse my health got, the wackier my jokes got.

By avoiding my new "reality" and not allowing myself to experience the pain, I probably didn't accept my "new normal" or transfer my emotional investment from my past physical, cognitive and emotional abilities and invest them in my new body, mind and spirit as quickly as I could have.

At the same time, I do believe that "humor is the best medicine." And if I hadn't joked, guffawed and made fun of my situation, my emotional recovery would have been even worse.

I'm living with these two contradictory thoughts in my head and, for the moment, grateful that I'm alive and ability to ponder them.

Notes

Preface

1. *Early Response Teams* ("ERT") of the United Methodist Committee on Relief ("UMCOR") are neither a first response group of emergency workers nor a recovery, rebuild or repair team. Their primary function is to provide "a caring Christian presence in the aftermath of a disaster." That having been said, the teams often help homeowners avoid further post-disaster damage by stabilizing their individual situations. This may including tarping damaged roofs, removing debris so they can enter and exit their homes, and cleaning or "mucking" out flooded homes.

   In addition, as presented in the "Train the Trainers" session of the UMCOR, North Central Jurisdiction's 2012 *Disaster Response Academy*, all ERTs are taught that disaster victims face these four stages/tasks in healing, emotionally, from a disaster. The stages are adapted from J. William Worden's "Four Tasks of Grief Model" as described in the *Grief Counseling and Grief Therapy: Handbook for the Mental Health Practitioner* (Springer Publishing Company, 1991).

Chapter 1

1. *The URL for the ABTA website is http://www.abta.org/index.cfm.*
2. *Pastor Dean is the Senior Pastor of the First United Methodist Church of Evanston. He's blessed with a superb intellect, a good nose for cooking, and a great eye for hanging drywall. Oh, and he's a pretty good preacher, too.*

Chapter 2

1. *C. F. Hathaway Company was a private manufacturer of shirts for men and boys, located in Waterville, Maine. It closed its Maine factory in 2002 making it the last major American shirt company to produce shirts in the United States. Hathaway is most famous for its "man with an eye patch" advertising campaign, which was created by*

Ogilvy & Mather in 1951. The "Hathaway Man" campaign was selected by Advertising Age as #22 on its list of the greatest ad campaigns of the 20th century.

Chapter 3

1. Stranger in a Strange Land is a Hugo award-winning science fiction novel by Robert A. Heinlein.
2. The phrase "...not no way, not no how..." is a quote from the movie, The Wizard of Oz, when a guard first refuses to let Dorothy and her entourage meet the wizard.
3. While working in Japan it took us awhile to catch on to the protocols for gift-giving. If you give a Japanese person a gift, they will give you a gift for giving them a gift. It can quickly become an arms-race of gift-giving if you don't cede the last gift to them.
4. I do not like horror movies, but this powerful visual has stuck with me. Should you be interested, you can it at http://www.moviegoods.com/movie_poster/hellraiser_1987.htm.

Chapter 4

1. Old Yeller is the name of a 1957 Walt Disney Productions film set in the Texas soon after the civil war ends. Old Yeller is the family dog that fights off a rabid wolf, and in so doing, gets rabies. The elder son is forced to kill the rabid dog. I remember it as a great coming-of-age movie.
2. I say "guy" in the Midwestern, ecumenical sense that everybody in the female gender can also be called "one of the guys."
3. Steve Magnino, who is often the smartest guy in the room, gave me this idea.
4. The Devil Wears Prada is a terrific film starring Meryl Streep and Ann Hathaway about the fashion industry and "life's choices." In the movie, Meryl Streep plays a tyrannical, manipulative and thoroughly unpleasant boss.
5. My dorky blue mask reminded me of the book, The Man in the Iron Mask by Alexandre Dumas. The book climactically concludes the epic adventures of the three Musketeers: Athos, Porthos, Aramis, and their friend D'Artagnan, how once invincible, meet their destinies. At this time, I was feeling like I was meeting my destiny and didn't like it one little bit.
6. Guy Fieri is the host of the Diners, Drive-ins and Dives Food Network TV show who uses the word "Bam" emphatically and often.

Chapter 5

1. Groundhog Day is a 1993 American comedy film directed by Harold Ramis, starring Bill Murray and Andie MacDowell. In the movie, Murray plays Phil Connors, an egocentric Pittsburgh TV weatherman who, during a hated assignment covering the annual Groundhog Day event in Punxsutawney, finds himself repeating the same day over and

over again. After indulging in hedonism and numerous suicide attempts, he begins to re-examine his life and priorities which enables him to escape the "do loop" in which he's caught.

2. According to the website "Phrase Finder", the "pros from Dover" is a slang term for outside consultants who are brought into a business to troubleshoot and solve problems. I vividly remember the term being used in the movie M*A*S*H*.

3. Patricia Anstett, "New Tools for Fixing Your Brain", Detroit Free Press, April 18, 2011

4. Slip 'n Slide is a toy manufactured by Wham-O. The toy is a long sheet of thin plastic, flanked lengthwise on one side by a heat-sealed tubular fold. The tube can be attached to any ordinary garden hose. Water runs through the tube and out small perforations, spraying onto the sliding surface. The Slip 'n Slide then becomes (guess what?) very slippery, enabling users to jump onto the plastic and slide the length of the sheet. We bought one and our kids had a great time with it for a least a day or two before becoming bored.

Chapter 6

1. According the online Urban Dictionary, "peeps" is short for "people" or "friends, close pals."

2. From the Wikipedia article: http://en.wikipedia.org/wiki/Gabrielle_Giffords.

3. CBS News website posting: http://www.cbsnews.com/8301-504763_162-20064258-10391704.html.

4. It's very important to defrost the skull because, otherwise, when inserted it would redefine the term, "brain freeze."

5. For the most part I've tried to call out the parts of this book that I've imagined or tried to re-create in a dramatic fashion to keep the narrative flow rolling smoothly. In contrast, I think the nurses' dialogue during my PIC line insertion is factually accurate, or actually factual, whichever makes the most grammatical sense.

6. The online postings of radiation treatment victims that I've read made me believe that my treatment was unusually easy. A conversation I had with a cancer victim who had weeks of every-other-day radiation treatments, treatments that sapped all her strength and were physically debilitating, has confirmed that suspicion.